Mobile Computing Solutions for Healthcare Systems

Edited by

Sivakumar R.

Department of Sensor and Biomedical Technology, School of Electronics Engineering, Vellore Institute of Technology, Vellore, India

Dimiter Velev

Department of Information Technology and Communications
The University of National and World Economy
Bulgaria

Basim Alhadidi

Department of Computer Information Systems
AlBalqa' Applied University Salt 19117,
Jordan

S. Vidhya

Department of Sensor and Biomedical Technology
Vellore Institute of Technology
Vellore
India

Sheeja V. Francis
Department of Electronics & Communication Engineering,
Jerusalem College of Engineering Chennai,Tamil Nadu,
India

&

B. Prabadevi
Department of Information Technology
School of Information Technology and Engineering
Vellore Institute of Technology,
Vellore
India

Mobile Computing Solutions for Healthcare Systems

Editors: Sivakumar R., Dimiter Velev, Basim Alhadidi, S. Vidhya,
Sheeja V. Francis and B. Prabadevi

ISBN (Online): 978-981-5050-59-2

ISBN (Print): 978-981-5050-60-8

ISBN (Paperback): 978-981-5050-61-5

First published in 2023.

Bentham Science Publishers Pte. Ltd.
80 Robinson Road #02-00
Singapore 068898
Singapore
Email: subscriptions@benthamscience.net

BENTHAM SCIENCE

CONTENTS

FOREWORD 1

Over the last decade, technological revolution has translated health care systems from its conventional form to the present computer / internet / mobile phone based formats. This paradigm shift has led to several advancements and challenges as well, which need scholarly deliberations. I am immensely pleased to find that this book provides such a platform. This book offers a comprehensive coverage of the wide spectrum of computing solutions available for mobile healthcare systems. It focuses on recent developments such as Artificial Intelligence, Machine Learning Methods, Medical Image Processing, Network Security and Antenna Design techniques, which may be integrated to build promising and secure m-Healthcare systems. Chapters on Smart Wearable Sensors and IoT based solutions for general remote health monitoring as well as their specific application during COVID pandemic are truly contemporary. I congratulate the editors for providing a platform for several researchers to showcase their research findings and achievements in the field of m-Healthcare. I am sure that this book will provide several insights and directions for further research in the area.

M. Sasikala
Department of Electronics & Communication Engineering
Anna University, Chennai
Tamilnadu
India

FOREWORD 2

The book presents the latest developments on integrating Artificial Intelligence and Machine Learning methods, medical image processing, advanced network security, and advanced antenna design techniques to bring Mobile Healthcare (M-Health) to new advanced, promising and secure M-Healthcare systems. The book aims to bring together scientists and practitioners from different professional fields to address several kinds of research and achievements in M-Healthcare, based on intelligent IoT and Machine Learning systems for personalized intelligent M-Healthcare and remote monitoring applications. The book will certainly be of special interest to a wide professional audience and it will give precious insights on how to effectively fight diseases with the newest technologies.

Dimitar Dimitrov
Rector of University of National and World Economy
Bulgaria

PREFACE

Mobile Health (M-Health) integrates the Internet of Things, mobile computing, medical image processing, medical sensor, and communications technology for mobile healthcare applications. Wireless Body Area Networks (WBANs) of intelligent sensors represent an emerging technology for system integration with great potential for unobtrusive ambulatory health monitoring during extended periods. However, system designers will have to resolve several issues, such as severe limitations of sensor weight and size necessary to improve user compliance, sensor resource constraints, intermittent availability of uplink connectivity, and reliability of transmission, security, and interoperability of different platforms. In addition, there are many challenges like Frequency Band Selection, Antenna Design, Channel Modelling, Energy-efficient hardware, Real-time connectivity over heterogeneous networks Security and Privacy, and others. With the WBAN placed on the patient body in rural areas and the mobile computing devices having the intelligence to acquire and process the data immediately, some of the issues like security and privacy are overcome. More intelligent processing is made available in handheld devices by building more facilities in the device software. This book focuses on recent developments in integrating AI, machine learning methods, medical image processing, advanced network security, and advanced antenna design techniques to bring M-Healthcare systems, leading to a new, promising, and secure M-Healthcare system. This book aims to bring together researchers and practitioners to address several types of research and achievements in the field of M-Healthcare-based intelligent IoT and Machine Learning based systems for personalized intelligent M-Healthcare and remote monitoring applications.

The book is organized into eleven chapters. A brief description of each of the chapters is as follows:

Chapter 1 identifies the existing challenges in the management of channel estimation methods for high-mobility 5G- OFDM systems for 5G. The chapter sets the scene for discussions presented by various authors. In particular, the chapter presented a new channel estimation method for high-mobility 5G- OFDM systems for 5G. Furthermore, the chapter proposed a scheme that is feasible for many current wireless OFDM communication systems.

Chapter 2 presents a novel short-term prediction method for COVID-19. The authors examine the understanding of some challenges and inaccurate predictions of the natural progression of COVID-19. The overall aim of the chapter is to propose a mobile health (M-Health) App and help the user to know the status of the pandemic state and act accordingly.

Chapter 3 presents intrusion detection in IoT-based health monitoring systems. The authors of this chapter implemented and compared the various algorithms on the BoT-IoT dataset and their performance measures.

Chapter 4 presents an analysis of issues and concerns in machine learning methods for intelligent healthcare. The authors provide an outline of the requesting circumstances, conduit, and methods of sharp well-being. A logical conduit of information handling is obliged for regular intelligent well-being, information securing, records preparing, insights dispersal, data security and privateness, and systems administration and processing advancements.

Chapter 5 presents the multi-factor authentication protocol based on electrocardiography signals for a mobile cloud computing environment. This chapter has addressed a proposal and a partial evaluation of a multi-modal protocol that uses three factors (password, IMSI, and biometric signals based on electrocardiograms) to provide mutual authentication to users and CSP.

Chapter 6 reviews the recent trends in the internet of things, challenges, and opportunities. The authors systematically review the analysis of IoT protection and privacy problems, current security strategies, and a list of open topics for potential study.

Chapter 7 discusses the robust medical image watermarking techniques for secure medical data transmission in the mobile healthcare system. Two Robust medical image watermarking techniques are discussed. In the first method, an intelligent-based robust medical image watermarking technique is considered using a genetic algorithm. In the second method, visual meaningful image encryption is discussed to overcome the visual attack.

Chapter 8 presents the smartphone-based real-time monitoring and forecasting of drinking water quality using LSTM and GRU in the IoT Environment. The authors show that analysis made using GRU is much faster than LSTM, whereas the prediction of LSTM is slightly more accurate than GRU. The proposed system produces accurate results and can be implemented in schools and other drinking water resources.

Chapter 9 presents the IoT-enabled crowd monitoring and control to avoid covid disease spread using CrowdNet and YOLO. The authors proposed two modules; a deep CNN CrowdNet people counting algorithm to detect the distance between humans in highly dense crowds and an IoT platform for sending information to the authorities whenever there is a violation. Image processing is carried out in two parts: extraction of frames from real-time videos using YOLO CV, and the second one is the processing of the frame to detect the number of people present in the crowd.

Chapter 10 presents a game-based neurorehabilitation technology to augment the motor activity of hemiparesis patients. The authors of this chapter proposed a method that involves the design of neurorehabilitation technology by developing game-based interventions to improve the motor activities of hemiparesis patients.

Chapter 11 proposes smart wearable sensor design techniques for mobile healthcare solutions. The authors of this chapter discuss the technological developments that have led to the clinical utility of smart wearable body sensors. The authors have highlighted the points in how smart wearable sensors can enhance the physician-patient relationship, promote remote monitoring techniques, and impact healthcare management and spending.

Sivakumar R.
Department of Sensor and Biomedical Technology
School of Electronics Engineering
Vellore Institute of Technology, Vellore, India

Dimiter Velev
Department of Information Technology and Communications
The University of National and World Economy, Bulgaria

Basim Alhadid
Department of Computer Information Systems
AlBalqa' Applied University Salt 19117, Jordan

S. Vidhya
Department of Sensor and Biomedical Technology
School of Electronics Engineering
Vellore Institute of Technology, Vellore, India

Sheeja V. Francis
Department of Electronics & Communication Engineering
Jerusalem College of Engineering, Pallikaranai, Chennai, India

B. Prabadevi
Department of Information Technology
School of Information Technology and Engineering
Vellore Institute of Technology, Vellore, India

List of Contributors

Adson F. da Rocha	Electrical Engineering Department, University of Brasilia (UnB), Brasilia-DF, Brazil Biomedical Engineering Graduate Program, University of Brasilia at Gama (FGA/UnB), Gama-GO, Brazil
Aswin Shriram T.	SASTRA Deemed University, India
B. Prathusha Laxmi	R.M.K. Engineering College, Chennai, India
B. Priyanka	Junior Research Fellow, VIT University, Chennai, India
B. Raghul	Associate Analys, ZIFO R & D Solutions, India
Bharathi N.	SRM Institute of Science and Technology, Vadapalani, Chenna, India
Brindha G.R.	SASTRA Deemed University, India
Cristiano J. Miosso	Biomedical Engineering Graduate Program, University of Brasilia at Gama (FGA/UnB), Gama-GO, Brazil
Eshita Suri	Vellore Institute of Technology, Vellore, Tamil Nadu, India
G. Valarmathi	Department of Electronics and Communication Engineering, Sri Sairam Institute of Technology, Chennai, Tamilnadu, India
Immanuel Rajkumar R.	Sathyabama Institute of Science and Technology, Chenna, India
J. Jeba Emilyn	Sona College of Technology, Salem-63600 Tamil Nadu, India
J. Sofia Bobby	Department of Biomedical Engineering, Jerusalem College of Engineering, Chennai-100, India
K. Kalaivani	Department of Electronics and Instrumentation Engineering, Easwari Engineering College, Chennai, Tamilnadu, India
K. Vijaya	SRM Institute of Science and Technology, Chennai, India
M.N. Ahil	Department of Information Technology, Kumaraguru College of Technology, Coimbatore, India
M. Prabu	National Institute of Technology Calicut, Kozhikode -673601, Kerala, India
N. Rajathi	Department of Information Technology, Kumaraguru College of Technology, Coimbatore, India
Paulo R. L. Gondim	Electrical Engineering Department, University of Brasilia (UnB), Brasilia-DF, Brazil
Poonguzhali S.	Sathyabama Institute of Science and Technology, Chennai, India
R. Nagarajan	Department of Electrical and Electronics Engineering, Gnanamani College of Technology, Tamilnadu, India
Rishiikeshwer B.S.	SASTRA Deemed University, India
S. Kannadhasan	Department of Electronics and Communication Engineering, Cheran College of Engineering, Tamilnadu, India
S. Priya	School of Computing, SASTRA Deemed University, Thanjavur, Tamilnadu, India
Sameer Ahamed R.	Vellore Institute of Technology, Vellore, Tamil Nadu, India

Sanjay Raju	SASTRA Deemed University, India
Santhi B.	School of Computing, SASTRA Deemed University, Thanjavur, Tamilnadu, India
Sathish Kumar D.	IFET college of Engineering, Gangarampalayam, India
Silas L. Albuquerque	Electrical Engineering Department, University of Brasilia (UnB), Brasilia-DF, Brazil
Srinija Ramichetty	Vellore Institute of Technology, Vellore, Tamil Nadu, India
Sujatha Rajkumar	Vellore Institute of Technology, Vellore, Tamil Nadu, India
T. Kalaiselvi	Department of Electronics and Instrumentation Engineering, EaswariEngineering College, Chennai, Tamilnadu, India
V. Murugan	Trichy Engineering College, Trichy-621132 Tamil Nadu, India
V. Subashini	Department of Electronics and Communication Engineering, Sri Sairam Institute of Technology, Chennai, Tamilnadu, India
V. Vanitha	Department of Information Technology, Kumaraguru College of Technology, Coimbatore, India

CHAPTER 1

An SDN Based WBAN using Congestion Control Routing Algorithm with Energy Efficiency

Poonguzhali S.[1,*], **Sathish Kumar D.**[2] and **Immanuel Rajkumar R.**[1]

[1] *Sathyabama Institute of Science and Technology, Chennai, India*

[2] *IFET College of Engineering, Gangarampalayam, India*

Abstract: The use of a Software-Defined Network (SDN) approach improves the control and management processes of the complex structured wireless sensor network. Also, it provides higher flexibility and a dynamic network structure. SDN is introduced to efficiently and opportunistically use the limited spectrum to minimize the spectrum scarcity issues. The LEACH protocol is self-organizing and is characterized as an adaptive clustering protocol that randomly distributes energy load among nodes. By using cluster heads and data aggregation, excessive energy consumption is avoided. SDN is often placed in an open environment and is susceptible to various attacks. The routing is based on multihop's flawless hauling range data transmission between the base station and cluster heads.The advantage of LEACH is that each node has the same probability of being a cluster head, which makes the energy efficiency of each node relatively balanced. Massive multiple-input multiple outputs (MIMO) play a polar role within the fifth generation (5G) wireless networks. However, its performance heavily depends on correct synchronization. Although timing offset (TO) can be avoided by applying orthogonal frequency division multiplexing (OFDM) with an adequate length of cyclic prefix (CP), carrier frequency offset (CFO) is still a challenging issue. Especially in the uplink of multiuser massive MIMO systems, CFO compensation can impose a substantial amount of computational complexity on the base station (BS) due to many BS antennas. However, to the best of our knowledge, no study looks into the joint estimation of CFOs and wireless channels in orthogonal frequency division multiplexing (OFDM) based massive MIMO systems. In this project, we propose a low-complexity CFO compensation technique to resolve this problem. In our paper, to traumatize this issue, we tend to propose a low-complexity frequency synchronization technique with high accuracy for the transmission of multiuser orthogonal-frequency-division multiplexing-based large MIMO systems. First, we propose a carrier frequency offset (CFO) estimation whose process complexity will increase linearly concerning the quantity of base station (BS) antennas. We then propose a joint CFO compensation technique that is performed when combining the received signals at the BS antennas. As a result, its machine complexity exceeds the number of BS antennas. As a third contribution, the impact of the joint CFO estimation error is studied, and it is tested that by applying our planned joint CFO compensation technique, the joint CFO

* **Corresponding author Poonguzhali S.:** Sathyabama Institute of Science and Technology, Chennai, India; Tel: 9176303408; E-mail: poornidp@gmail.com

Sivakumar R., Dimiter Velev, Basim Alhadidi, S. Vidhya, Sheeja V. Francis and B. Prabadevi (Eds.)

estimation error causes a continuing section shift solely. We tend to propose an algorithm to expeditiously calculate and take away the estimation error. Our simulation results testify to the effectiveness of our planned synchronization technique. As it is incontestable, our planned synchronization technique results in a bit of error rate performance that is the one for an asynchronous system. This leads to a considerable saving in the computational cost of the receiver. Numerical results are presented to verify the performance of our proposed joint CFO compensation technique and to investigate its computational complexity.

Keywords: Congestion avoidance, Energy-efficiency, Enhanced multi-objective spider monkey optimization, Remote health monitoring, Software-defined network, Specific, Temperature-aware routing, The absorption rate, Wireless body area network.

INTRODUCTION

Driven by the fast step-up of the wireless capability necessities obligatory by advanced multimedia system applications (*e.g.*, ultrahigh-definition video, videogame, *etc.*), and because of the dramatically increasing demand for user access needed for the Internet of Things (IoT), the fifth-generation (5G) networks face challenges in terms of supporting giant-scale heterogeneous information traffic. 5G-OFDM, which has been recently projected for the third-generation partnership project involving long-term evolution advanced (3GPP-LTE-A), constitutes a promising technology for addressing the said challenges in 5G networks by accommodating many users among similar orthogonal resource blocks. By doing this, therefore, important information measure potency improvement is often earned over standard orthogonal multiple-access (OMA) techniques. These various actual analyzers dedicate substantial research contributions to the current field. In this context, we offer a comprehensive summary of state-of-the-art power domain multiplexing-aided 5G-OFDM, with a focus on the theoretical 5G-OFDM principles, multiple-antenna-aided 5G-OFDM design, on the interaction between 5G-OFDM and cooperative transmission, on the resource management of 5G- OFDM, the beingness of 5G-OFDM with alternative rising potential 5G techniques and the comparison with alternative 5G-OFDM variants. We highlight the main advantages of power-domain multiplexing 5G-OFDM compared to alternative existing OFDM techniques. We summarize the challenges of existing research contributions of 5G-OFDM and supply potential solutions. Finally, we provide some design guidelines for 5G-OFDM systems and determine promising analysis opportunities for the long run.

Multiuser Detection

We will solely support K users if we tend to use orthogonal K-chips. However, we will have more users once non-orthogonal m -sequences are victimized within the spirit of 5G-OFDM. Multiple-access interference (MAI) limits the capability and performance of CDMA systems. Whereas the MAI caused by one officious user is tiny, the system becomes interference restricted primarily because the variety of interferers or their power will increase. MUD exploiting the information of each the spreading code associated temporal order (and probably amplitude and phase) information of multiple users has been thought to be an efficient strategy of raising the system capability. Various MUD algorithms, such as the optimal maximum-likelihood sequence estimation, turbo cryptography, matched filter SIC, and parallel interference cancellation (PIC), are designed to scale back the MAI at an inexpensive complexness value. Moreover, some recently developed joint detection techniques for downlink systems are based on single-antenna interference cancellation (SAIC) receivers. This technique depends on either maximum-likelihood detection or pre-detection processing, instead of IC techniques. This development is attributed to the fact that joint detection has also been developed for asynchronous networks [1]. As an additional advance, the proposed SAIC technique has had successful field trial results in the GSM era to suppress the downlink inter-cell interference.

Interference Cancellation

The multiuser IC techniques may be divided into two main classes, particularly pre-interference cancelation (pre-IC) and post-interference cancellation (post-IC). More specifically, pre-IC techniques are utilized at the facet side by suppressing the interference by pre-coding approaches like the famous dirty paper coding (DPC) upon exploiting the knowledge of the channel state information (CSI) at the transmitter. By contrast, the post-IC techniques are usually used on the receiver side to cancel the interference. The post-IC approach can be further divided into two categories, which are parallel and serial. If we carry out accurate power control to ensure that all received signals are similar, PIC outperforms SIC. By contrast, SIC works better when the received powers are different because the strongest user's signal can be detected first. The detected bit is the re-modulate, and its interference is deducted from the received signal. Repeating this action in a sequential order gives us the clean weakest signal. It is worth noting that in addition to the performance *versus* complexity tradeoff, there are also a variety of other tradeoffs between PIC and SIC. There are some recent IC techniques.

EXISTING SYSTEM

A simple self-polarization-stabilization technique for the wavelength-division-multiplexed passive optical network implemented with reflective semiconductor optical amplifiers (RSOAs) and self-homodyne coherent receivers. A 45-degree Faraday rotator is placed in front of the RSOA in the optical network unit. The state of polarization of the upstream signal becomes orthogonal to that of the linearly polarized seed light at the input of the coherent receiver regardless of the birefringence in the transmission link. Thus, we can achieve the polarization stability of the upstream signal at the input of the coherent receiver. We first implement a self-homodyne receiver using the proposed self-polarization-stabilization technique and measure its sensitivity using 2.5-Gb/s binary phase-shift keying signals in the laboratory. The result shows an excellent receiver sensitivity of dBm. We also confirm the efficacy of the proposed technique in the transmission experiment over a 68-km long link partially composed of installed (buried and aerial) fibers. No significant degradation in the receiver sensitivity is observed during the 10-h experiment despite the large polarization fluctuations in these installed fibers.

There has been growing interest in the long-reach passive optical network (PON) due to the possibility of reducing the cost per subscriber by increasing the coverage of the central office (CO) [1 - 7]. In particular, the long-reach hybrid wavelength-division-multiplexed (WDM)/time-division-multiplexed (TDM) PON appears to be the most promising solution for drastically increasing the number of subscribers covered by a CO [2 - 7]. In the case of using a remote optical amplifier for the compensation of the losses occurring in the transmission fiber and remote node (RN), it is difficult to realize the WDM PON in loopback configuration (which is needed for the colorless operation) since the system's performance can be seriously degraded by the effect of Rayleigh backscattering. Recently proposed and demonstrated a long-reach WDM PON in loopback configuration using reflective semiconductor optical amplifiers (RSOAs) and self-homodyne coherent receivers. This network is entirely "passive" since there is no need to use the remote amplifier in the outside plant. In addition, to enhance its cost-effectiveness, we realize the coherent receiver by using a portion of the seed light (used to generate the upstream signal) as a local oscillator (LO) and an inexpensive three-fiber coupler as a 120 optical hybrid. However, for practical deployment, this coherent receiver still requires the use of the polarization-diversity technique (or the polarization-tracking technique) [6 - 10], which may be too expensive for use in the cost-sensitive access network. This paper proposes the self-polarization-stabilization technique for use in the long-reach RSOA-based WDM PON implemented with self-homodyne coherent receivers. To achieve the upstream signal at the input of the coherent receiver's input, we place a 45-degree

Faraday rotator (FR) in front of the RSOA in the optical network unit (ONU).

The state-of-polarization (SOP) of the upstream signal becomes orthogonal to that of the linearly polarized seed light at the input of the coherent receiver located at the CO, regardless of the birefringence in the transmission link. Thus, we can detect the upstream signal using a single-polarization coherent receiver instead of the expensive polarization-diversity receiver., We implement a 2.5-Gb/s WDM PON using RSOAs and self- homodyne coherent receivers. The sensitivity of the self-homodyne receiver is measured to be dBm (at bit error ratio). To evaluate the effectiveness of the proposed self-polarization-stabilization technique, we also perform a long-term BER measurement by using a 68-km-long transmission link composed of both buried and aerial fibers. No significant degradation in the receiver sensitivity is observed during our 10-h experiment despite the large polarization fluctuations in the installed fiber.

Exhaustive Search Method for Channel Estimation For OFDM

OFDM is a channel access method for shared medium networks. It allows several users to share the same frequency channel by dividing the signal into different time slots. The users transmit in rapid succession, one after the other, each using its time slot. The existing system considers energy-efficient transmissions for OFDM networks in which the secondary users coexist with the primary users. We want to optimize the proper time allocations and the beam-forming vectors for the secondary users, to minimize the total energy consumption of the secondary users while satisfying secondary users' rate requirements and the primary receivers' received interference constraints [3]. The joint time scheduling and beam-forming optimization are non-convex and are often highly complex to solve. Fortunately, we show that the optimal time allocation and the optimal beam-forming vectors can be found very efficiently in polynomial time through a proper decomposition.

DISADVANTAGES OF EXISTING SYSTEM

• Elimination of ISI causes Inter-Channel Interference (ICI).

• The BER performance is not improved. It leads to a decrement in SNR.

• Tight Synchronization between users is required in the receiver. It leads to time latency.

• Co-channel interference occurs.

• Dealing with this is more complex in OFDM than in CDMA. Static channel allocation with advanced coordination among adjacent base stations.

• The OFDM signal has a noise-like amplitude with a very large dynamic range. Therefore, it requires RF power amplifiers with a high peak-to-average power ratio [11].

• It is more sensitive to carrier frequency offset and drifts than single carrier systems due to the DFT leakage.

PROPOSED METHODOLOGY

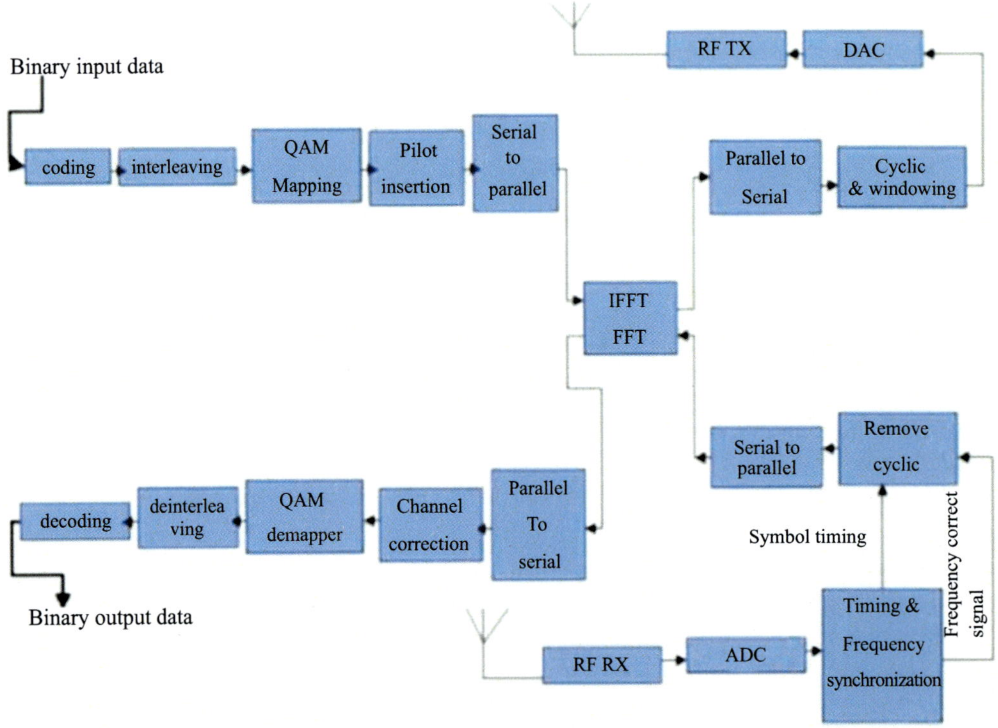

Fig. (1). Block diagram of the proposed system.

The proposed system is done over additive white Gaussian noise (AWGN) and impulsive noise (which is produced in broadband transmission) channels which is shown in Fig. (**1**). In this paper, Bit, the Error Rate performance of the 5G-OFDM 16-QAM System over the Rayleigh fading channel is analyzed. 5G-OFDM is orthogonal frequency division multiplexing to reduce inter-symbol interference problems. The equalization algorithm is a Normalized LMMSE equalizer. Finally, simulations of 5G-OFDM signals are carried out with Rayleigh faded signals to understand the effect of channel fading and to obtain the optimum value of Bit Error Rate (BER) and Signal to noise ratio (SNR) [4]. The channel distortion is addressed by a deep learning model that is first trained offline using the data generated from simulation based on channel statistics and then used for recovering the online transmitted data directly.

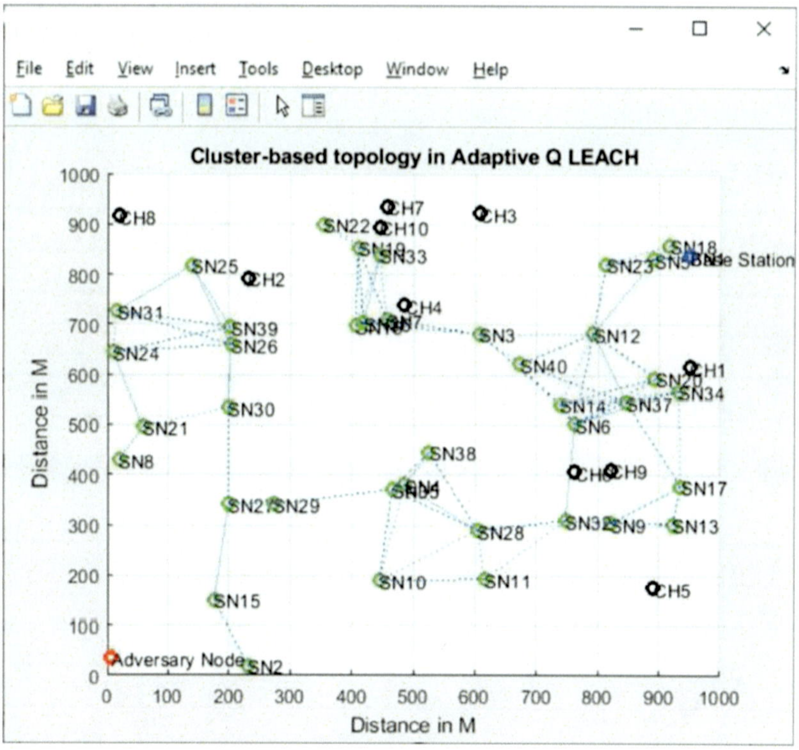

Fig. (2). Cluster-based topology in adaptive Q LEACH.

The deep learning-based approach can address channel distortion from the proposed system and detect the transmitted symbols with performance comparable to the linear minimum mean square error (LMMSE) estimator. The proposed approach adopts the repetitive signal structure of 5G-OFDM, such as the cyclic prefix (5G), which can be used for synchronization purposes. The originally derived ML estimation results in a high computational cost; therefore, after gaining insights into the log-likelihood (LL) function, we further design an algorithm with reduced complexity. Furthermore, the deep learning-based approach is more robust than conventional methods when fewer training pilots are used, the cyclic prefix (5G) is omitted, and nonlinear clipping noise exists.

RESULTS AND DISCUSSION

The operation of LEACH consists of several rounds with two phases in each round. The working of Q-LEACH starts with the formation of clusters based on the received signal strength [5]. SDN is a new network architecture model that gathers the advances of statements previously mentioned. It separates the control base station and database station in network devices to enable a Programmable behavior removing the rigidity of secured protocols. Tables **1** and **2** listed the simulated SNR for various BER values. Fig. (**2**) shows the LEACH methods for various differentiating distances.

Table 1. 5G SDN LMMSE.

BER	SNR in dB
0.0019	0
0.0013	2
0.0008	4
0.0004	6
0.0001	8
0.0000	10
0.0000	12
0.0000	14
0	16
0	18
0	20

Table 2. 5G SDN.

BER	SNR in dB
0.2822	0
0.1954	0
0.1178	0
0.056	0
0.0187	1
0.0034	2
0.0003	3
0	4
0	5
0	6
0	7

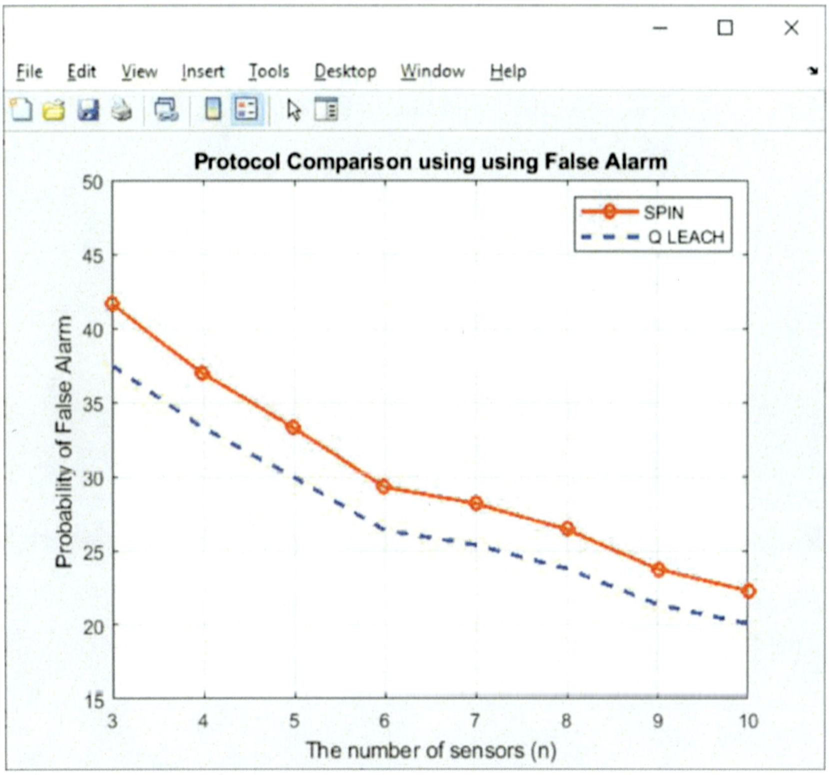

Fig. (3). Protocol comparison using false alarm.

The false alarm should be minor for energy-efficient protocol. As shown in the Fig. (**3**), the Q LEACH protocol gives low false alarms compared to the SPIN – (Sensor Protocol for Information *via* Negotiation) protocol.

The number of packets is sent to the base station for the SPIN protocol is illustrated in Fig. (**4**). The data rate is a term to denote the transmission speed or the number of bits per second transferred [6]. The valuable data rate for the user is usually less than the actual data rate transported on the network.

In Fig. (**5**), the number of packets sent to the base station is high for the Q-LEACH protocol. It is inferred that, the number of packets sent to Base station nodes [7] of Q LEACH is better than others. Fig. (**6**) shows the energy efficiency for different WSN.

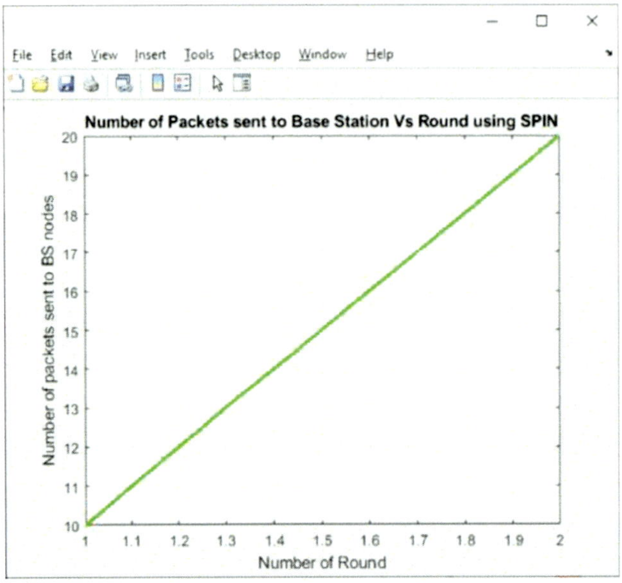

Fig. (4). Number of packets sent to base station *vs.* round using spin.

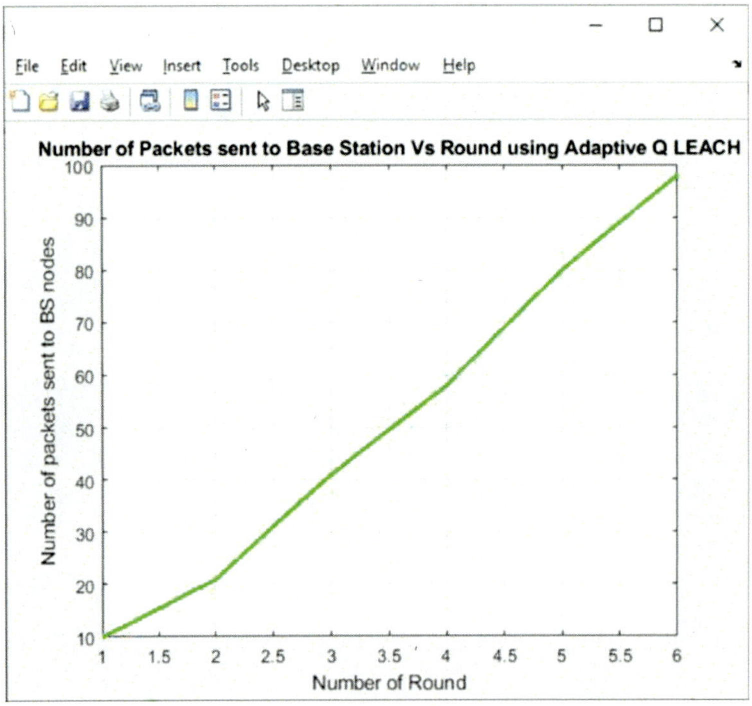

Fig. (5). Number of packets sent to base station *vs.* round using adaptive Q LEACH.

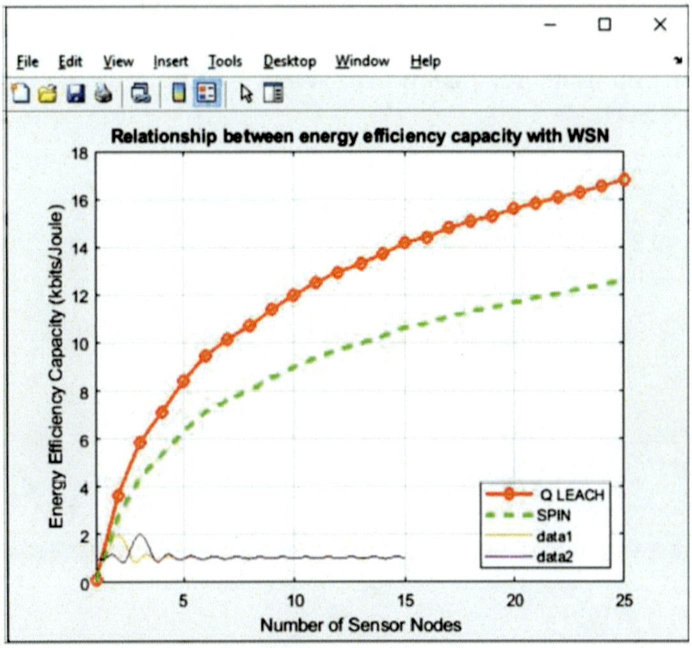

Fig. (6). Relationship between energy efficiency capacity with WSN.

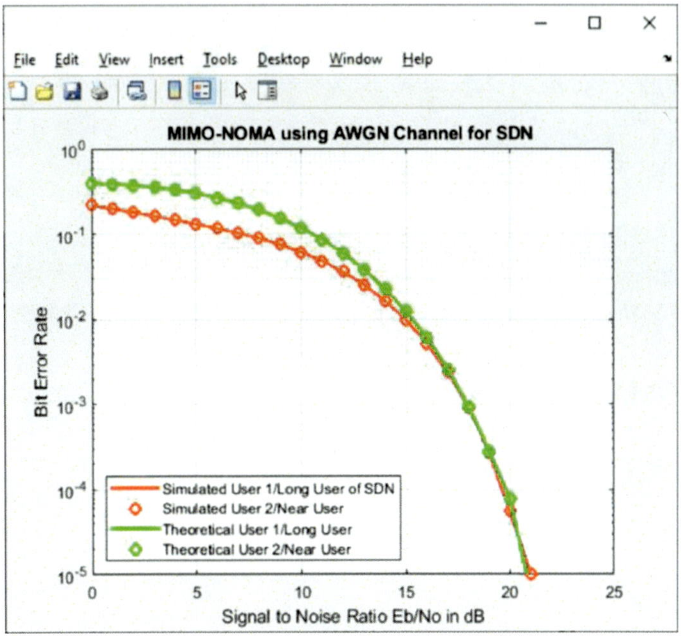

Fig. (7). MIMO-NOMA using AWGN channel for SDN.

The MIMO NOMA is implemented for AWGN (Additive White Gaussian Noise) channel for SDN. The Bit Error Rate *vs.* Signal to Noise Ratio in dB is plotted [8]. The simulation for users for different distances (long and Near) is plotted for various users of SDN.

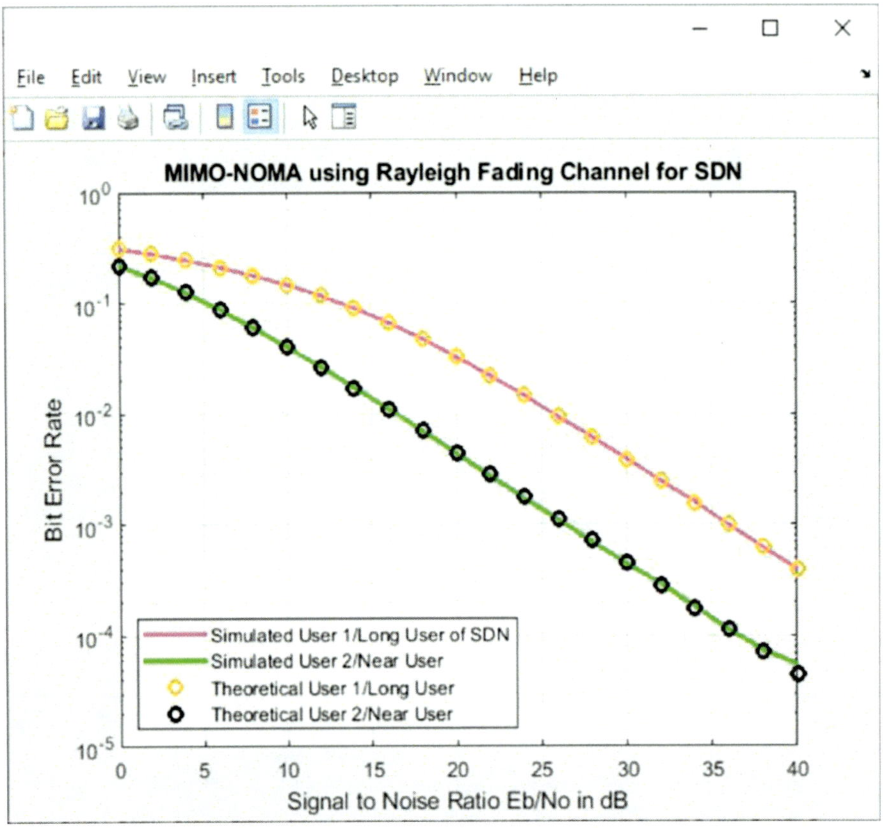

Fig. (8). MIMO- NOMA using Rayleigh Fading Channel for SDN.

The MIMO NOMA is implemented for the Rayleigh fading channel for SDN. Fig. (7) illustrated the impact of BER for AWGN channel. The Bit Error Rate *vs.* Signal to Noise Ratio in dB using Rayleigh model is plotted in Fig. (**8**). The simulation for users for different distances (long and Near) is plotted for various SDN users [9].

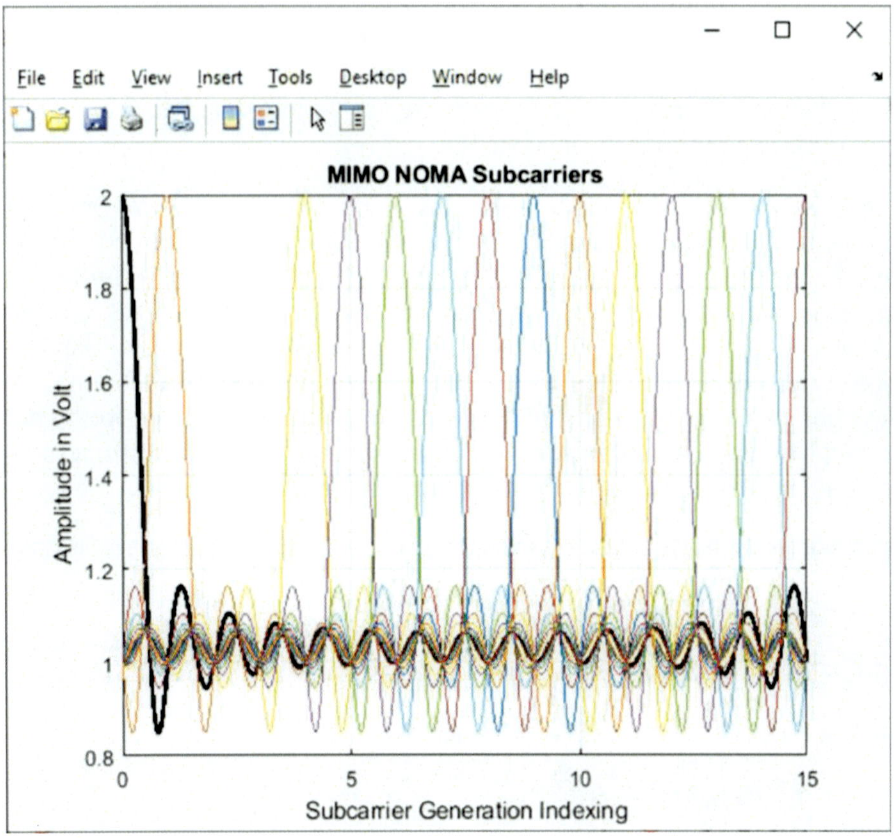

Fig. (9). MIMO NOMA subcarriers.

The MIMO NOMA is implemented for the Rayleigh fading channel for SDN. The Bit Error Rate *vs.* Signal to Noise Ratio in dB is plotted. The MIMO NOMA is implemented in the proposed methodology for SDN and analyzed for different NOMA subcarriers is illustrated in Fig. (**9**). Nonorthogonal multiple access (NOMA) principles emerge as a solution to improve spectral efficiency while allowing some degree of multiple access interference at receivers [10]. In this tutorial-style paper, we target providing a unified model for NOMA, including uplink and downlink transmissions, along with the extensions to multiple inputs multiple outputs, and cooperative communication scenarios in SDN.

CONCLUSION

This work presented a new channel estimation method for high-mobility 5G-OFDM systems for 5G. The proposed channel model channel reduces the estimation complexity by utilizing the position information [12]. The proposed algorithm jointly designs the pilot symbol and the placement to minimize the system's average coherence. Simulation results demonstrate that the proposed method performs better than existing channel estimation methods over high-mobility channels. Furthermore, the proposed scheme is feasible for many current wireless OFDM communication systems.

The wireless network modeling and simulation are implemented for communicating wireless data. The data mobility is improved in wireless communication by improving SNR and maximizing the system's throughput. The reduction in path loss and BER criteria is used to establish the ongoing call without dropping by keeping handoff, and the probability of establishing a new call could not be blocked due to a momentary lack of an idle channel. The 5G wireless network is used to provide secured communication by properly detecting intrusion [13]. The QoS is improved by calculating various parameters to prove the accurate implementation of the proposed system.

CONSENT FOR PUBLICATION

Not applicable.

CONFLICT OF INTEREST

The author declares no conflict of interest, financial or otherwise.

ACKNOWLEDGEMENTS

The authors, Aakanchha Jain and Santosh K. Behera are thankful to former Director, NIPER-A for providing necessary literature searching facilities.

REFERENCES

[1] P. Schniter, "Low-complexity equalization of OFDM in doubly selective channels", *IEEE Trans. Signal Process.,* vol. 52, no. 4, pp. 1002-1011, 2004. [http://dx.doi.org/10.1109/TSP.2004.823503]

[2] O.B. Karimi, J. Liu, and C. Wang, "Seamless wireless connectivity for multimedia services in high-speed trains", *IEEE J. Sel. Areas Comm.,* vol. 30, no. 4, pp. 729-739, 2012. [http://dx.doi.org/10.1109/JSAC.2012.120507]

[3] W.U. Bajwa, A.M. Sayeed, and R. Nowak, "Sparse multipath channels: Modeling and estimation", In: *Proc. IEEE Digit. Signal Process.* Educ.Workshop, 2009, pp. 320-325.

[4] W.U. Bajwa, J. Haupt, A.M. Sayeed, and R. Nowak, "Compressed channel sensing: A new approach to estimating sparse multipath channels", *Proc. IEEE,* vol. 98, no. 6, pp. 1058-1076, 2010. [http://dx.doi.org/10.1109/JPROC.2010.2042415]

[5] S. Poonguzhali, "A Non-Invasive multi-faced problem-solving tool in a Dynamic sensor network for Pediatric Diabetes with Fall Detection", In: *2nd International Conference on Power and Embedded Drive Control (ICPEDC)*Chennai, India, 2019, pp. 493-498. [http://dx.doi.org/10.1109/ICPEDC47771.2019.9036551]

[6] W. U. Bajwa, A. M. Sayeed, and R. Nowak, “Learning sparse doubly selective channels,” In: *Proc. 46th Annu. Allerton Conf. Commun.*, ControlComput., Sep. 2008, pp. 575–582. [http://dx.doi.org/10.1109/ALLERTON.2008.4797610]

[7] S. Sung, and D. Brady, "Spectral spatial equalization for OFDM in time-varying frequency-selective multipath channels", *Proc. IEEEWorkshopSensor Array Multichannel Signal Process.,* pp. 434-438, 2000.

[8] S. Poonguzhali, "Wireless Sensor Network with a Novel Key Distribution for Improved Four-Tier Network Security", *Res. J. Pharm. Biol. Chem. Sci.*, vol. 6, no. 4, pp. 319-327, 2015 [RJPBCS].

[9] Y. Mostofi, and D.C. Cox, "ICI mitigation for pilot-aided OFDM mobile systems", *IEEE Trans. Wirel. Commun.,* vol. 4, no. 2, pp. 765-774, 2005. [http://dx.doi.org/10.1109/TWC.2004.840235]

[10] H. Hijazi, and L. Ros, "Polynomial estimation of the time-varying multipath gain with intercarrier interference mitigation in OFDM systems", *IEEE Trans. Vehicular Technol.,* vol. 58, no. 1, pp. 140-151, 2009. [http://dx.doi.org/10.1109/TVT.2008.923653]

[11] Xiaoli Ma, G.B. Giannakis, and S. Ohno, "Optimal training for block transmissions over doubly selective wireless fading channels", *IEEE Trans. Signal Process.,* vol. 51, no. 5, pp. 1351-1366, 2003. [http://dx.doi.org/10.1109/TSP.2003.810304]

[12] S. Poonguzhali, "Rekha Chakravarthy. Performance improvisation using IOT based sensor network in telemedicine assistance by electrocardiogram signal analysis for diabetes healthcare", *Biomedicine (Taipei),* vol. 40, no. 1, pp. 83-88, 2020.

[13] Z. Tang, R.C. Cannizzaro, G. Leus, and P. Banelli, "Pilot-assisted time-varying channel estimation for OFDM systems", *IEEE Trans. Signal Process.,* vol. 55, no. 5, pp. 2226-2238, 2007. [http://dx.doi.org/10.1109/TSP.2007.893198]

CHAPTER 2

COVID-19 - Novel Short Term Prediction Methods

Sanjay Raju[1], Rishiikeshwer B.S.[1], Aswin Shriram T.[1], Brindha G.R.[1,*], Santhi B.[1,*] and **Bharathi N.[2,*]**

[1] *School of Computing, SASTRA Deemed to be University, Thanjavur, Tamilnadu, India*

[2] *SRM Institute of Science and Technology, Vadapalani, Chennai, India*

Abstract: The recent outbreak of Severe Acute Respiratory Syndrome Corona Virus (SARS-CoV-2), also called COVID-19, is a major global health problem due to an increase in mortality and morbidity. The virus disturbs the respirational process of a human being and is highly spreadable. The current distressing COVID-19 pandemic has caused heavy financial crashing and the assets and standards of the highly impacted countries being compromised. Therefore, prediction methods should be devised, supporting the development of recovery strategies. To make accurate predictions, understanding the natural progression of the disease is very important.

The developed novel mathematical models may help the policymakers and government control the infection and protect society from this pandemic infection. Due to the nature of the data, the uncertainty may lead to an error in the estimation. In this scenario, the uncertainty arises due to the dynamic rate of change based on time in the infectious count because of the different stages of lockdowns, population density, social distancing, and many other reasons concerning demography. The period between exposure to the virus and the first symptom of infection is large compared to other viruses. It is mandatory to follow the infected persons.

The exposure needs to be controlled to prevent the spreading in the long term, and the infected people must be in isolation for the above-mentioned period to avoid short-term infections. Officials need to know about the long-term scenario as well as the short-term for policymaking. Many studies are focusing on long-term forecasting using mathematical modelling. For the short-term prediction, this paper proposed two algorithms: 1) to predict next-day count from the past 2 days data irrespective of population size with less error rate and 2) to predict the next M days based on the deviation of the rate of change in previous N-days active cases.

The proposed methods can be adopted by government officials, researchers, and medical professionals by developing a mobile application. So that they can use it

* **Corresponding authors Brindha, G.R., Santhi, B. and Bharathi, N.:** SASTRA Deemed University, India and SRM Institute of Science and Technology, Vadapalani, Chennai, India; Tel: 9487755985, 9443079380 and 9566039944; E-mails: brindha.gr@ict.sastra.edu, shanthi@cse.sastra.edu and bharathn2@srmist.edu.in

Sivakumar R., Dimiter Velev, Basim Alhadidi, S. Vidhya, Sheeja V. Francis and B. Prabadevi (Eds.)

whenever and wherever necessary. The mobile health (M-Health) App. helps the user to know the status of the pandemic state and act accordingly.

Keywords: COVID-19, Error rate, India, Short term prediction, Spreading rate.

INTRODUCTION

COVID-19 dataset has 3 confirmed cases till Feb 2020 in India. From March 2020, the spreading started, and at the end of June 2020, the total confirmed count reached 400,000. The Indian health care system is handled by both government and private sectors. The people with symptoms are approaching both types of hospitals. They have to plan for infrastructure, manpower, and medical resources. The major focus is to be on rapid testing, diagnosis, availability of trained respiratory therapists, Intensive Care Unit staff, beds, test kits, *etc.* Planning is needed for rationing healthcare resources, which is inevitable for the assurance of consistent allocation. To provide full-fledged medical care with a 1.3 billion population and scarce resources, short-term planning is necessary, along with long-term forecasting. Even developed countries with abundant wealth and health care resources cannot manage the pandemic consequences and must evaluate how the available resources can be utilized rationally, reasonably, and effectively.

Many researchers predicted the count and flattened curve based on the SIR (Susceptible, Infected and Recovered) model, which was useful for making many decisions and preventive measures [1 - 4]. Stochastic and deterministic models can help find the infected size with dynamics over time. The Kermack-McKendrick model is governed by SIR and SEIR (Susceptible, Exposed, Infected, and Recovered) models, and it employs the infection age and structured assumption from 1927 [5]. If an exposed individual gets attached to the pathogen, he may become infected. An individual who is exposed to the pathogen through contact can also act as a carrier. The latent period is defined as the time for the infected person (host) to act as a carrier who can transmit pathogens to other people *via* contact. The incubation period is a period between being exposed to the pathogen and the onset of symptoms of the disease. It can also be defined as the time required for the pathogen to multiply itself to a level in the host to produce symptoms or laboratory evidence. The other features are incidence and prevalence. Incidence is defined as the number of individuals who were infected during a specified interval of time. Sometimes this number can also be divided by the total population. The prevalence is the number of people who have the disease at a specific time. This can also be divided by the total population [6, 7]. SIR and SEIR are standard epidemic models which predict the average number of cases or deaths during the outbreak [8, 9].

The expected number of secondary cases produced by a single infected case in a susceptible population is known as the reproduction number, which is related to daily impact. Many researchers studied this reproduction number since it varies based on country population size, lockdown status, and other parameters [10, 11]. For comparing the predicted values of existing studies, the actual values are taken from www.worldometers.info [12]. Kotwal *et al.* surveyed the COVID-19 studies and concluded a strong relationship between short-term predictions and uncertainty in long-term prediction [13].

The cause for uncertainty is the varying rate of change in cases. Nathaniel S. Barlow and Steven J. Weinstein found the advantage in deriving the analytic nature of the asymptotic approximation. They suggested that the model parameters were extracted through least squares or similar methods without the requirement for an embedded numerical scheme [14]. Another author focused on undetected persons and various infectious cases in hospitals. They analyzed china's COVID-19 data. The proposed model predicted the cases. The differences between the model predicted and the original were very less. This analysis gave an opinion to the policymakers [15]. Duccio Fanelli and Francesco Piazza applied nonlinear fitting and predicted the flattened curve for Italy with the detail that the peak in Italy would be around Mar 21st, 2020 and active count about 26000 (not including recovered and dead). Death counts at the end of the epidemics would be about 18,000 [16]. But 21-Mar, 2020 was not the peak (Apr 20th, 2020 was the peak day), and the infected count on that day was 53,528. Still (19th June 2020), it is not the end of the pandemic, and the death count is 34,514. Another study discussed that the isolation of the affected persons influences the spread of COVID-19. They applied numerical simulation to estimate the end time of the outbreaks [17]. Maleki *et al.* applied time series analysis and showed that the predicted cumulative world infected count and cured count were closer to the actual count [18].

Long short-term memory and deep learning were applied to predict the future cases of COVID-19 in Canada and other countries. The prediction on 28-Apr, 2020 was around 22,000 confirmed cases [19]. But the actual count on that day was 50,026. For the short duration, the RMSE value of 51.46 is less, but if the April month prediction is checked against the actual count, then for the LSTM model, the error will be more. From these studies and analysis, is it possible to predict the next day or week count that is closer to the actual? To solve this, the paper proposed two algorithms to predict the next day count from the two previous days, and predict the next M days count from the Previous N-days. The purpose of the short-term prediction is to plan the immediate requirement of beds, ventilators, test equipment, test plan, social distancing control, *etc.*

The Hurdles in Predicting COVID-19

• The exact count of people having immunity and mobility of people is unknown.

• Though people are safe at home, how careful are they handling things from outside? - cannot be computed by numeric values.

• Though social distancing is maintained in a commonplace, if the infected person passes the infection, say to an object, and when a non-infected person comes in contact with that object within the lifetime of that virus, the chance of spreading is more. This cannot be computed exactly.

• The existing prediction algorithms predicted a higher error rate, since earlier days, the infected count values were less, and the day-by-day increase also did not maintain uniformity.

Materials and Methods

The proposed two algorithms are:

• *Next-Day Prediction* - Using the average of the impact of the previous three days' values to predict next-day cases.

• *M-Days Prediction* - Using the Standard Deviation (SD) of the rate of change of previous N-days to predict the next M days cases.

Novel Next Day Prediction Method

The next-day prediction is based on the previous three days active count (A), which is only infected. The recovered cases (R) and death count (D) are not included in the active count. Exposure of the population of people to the pandemic infection varies due to the different stages of lockdown and restrictions followed at different locations. So, the proposed calculation does not consider the population but concentrates on the current infected cases and the 2 previous days to predict the count for tomorrow.

Where,

$$\textit{Next\_Day\_Count (NDC)} = (y_{mean} * A_{tod}) + A_{tod}$$

$$\textit{Where } y_{mean} = (y_{yst} + y_{tod}) / 2 ,$$

$$y_{yst} = x_{yst} / A_{yst} \quad \textit{Similarly,} \quad y_{tod} = x_{tod} / A_{tod} \quad \textit{and}$$

$$x_{yst} = A_{yst} - A_{dby} \quad \textit{and} \quad x_{tod} = A_{tod} - A_{yst}$$

x is the daily count and **y** is the daily impact on infection. **dby, yst** and **tod** are the days before yesterday, yesterday and today.

After substitution,

$$NDC = \frac{1}{2A_{yst}}\left(x_{yst}A_{tod} + x_{dby}A_{yst} + A_{tod}A_{yst}\right)$$

Finally, after generalizing,

$$NDC_{day\_i+1} = \frac{1}{2A_{day\_i-1}}\left(x_{day\_i-1}A_{day\_i} + x_{day\_i-2}A_{day\_i-1} + A_{day\_i}A_{day\_i-1}\right)$$

The above count is for active cases.

Similarly, for recovered cases and death cases, the corresponding count is substituted.

For Recovered cases:

$$NDC_{day\_i+1} = \frac{1}{2R_{day\_i-1}}\left(x_{day\_i-1}R_{day\_i} + x_{day\_i-2}R_{day\_i-1} + R_{day\_i}R_{day\_i-1}\right)$$

For Death cases:

$$NDC_{day\_i+1} = \frac{1}{2D_{day\_i-1}}\left(x_{day\_i-1}D_{day\_i} + x_{day\_i-2}D_{day\_i-1} + D_{day\_i}D_{day\_i-1}\right)$$

Though the above equations are illustrated in the following example. Fig. (**1**) explains the process of the proposed method.

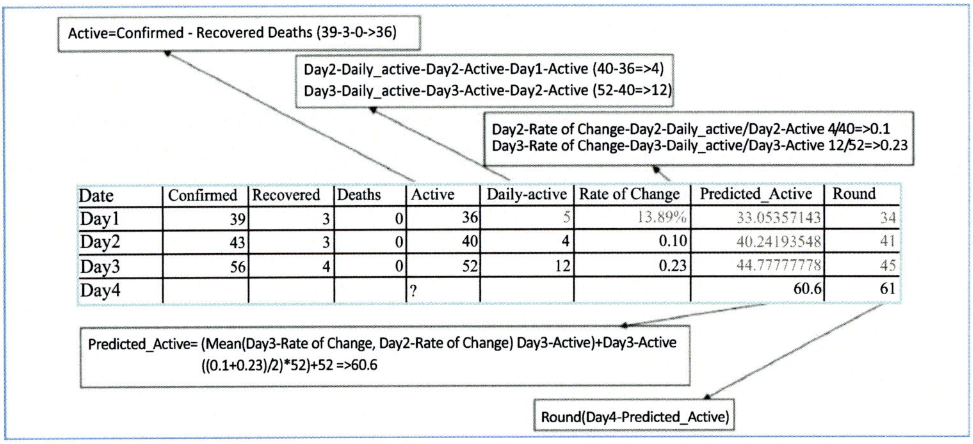

Date	Confirmed	Recovered	Deaths	Active	Daily-active	Rate of Change	Predicted_Active	Round
Day1	39	3	0	36	5	13.89%	33.05357143	34
Day2	43	3	0	40	4	0.10	40.24193548	41
Day3	56	4	0	52	12	0.23	44.77777778	45
Day4				?			60.6	61

Fig. (1). Sample process of the proposed next-day prediction mechanism.

Novel M Days Prediction Method

The M Days prediction method is applied to predict the active cases count for the Next M days. The same method can be used to forecast recovered and death cases for the next M days. This paper analyses the performance of the M days prediction method by predicting the 25 days active cases. M-Days prediction method uses the SD of the rate of change of active cases to predict N+1 to N+M days (M days). The M-Days prediction method is explained below and the implementation of this algorithm includes three stages: 1) SD Computation 2) Prediction Computation 3) Error rate Computation.

The N-days data is calculated before predicting the next M days by using the given equations which are already discussed in the next day prediction section.

$y_{yst} = x_{yst} / A_{yst}$ ***Similarly,*** $y_{tod} = x_{tod} / A_{tod}$ ***and***

$x_{yst} = A_{yst} - A_{dby}$ ***and*** $x_{tod} = A_{tod} - A_{yst}$

//SD Computation

Sample_Endday_Impact (SEI) $= day\_i - 1$

$Y = 0$ ***(Total change for N days)***

$Y = \sum_{i=1}^{n} y_{day\_i}$

$Y_{mean} = Y/n$ ***(Mean change)***

$S = \sum_{i=1}^{n} (y_{day\_i} - Y_{mean})^2$

Deviation (SD) $= \sqrt{S/SEI}$

//Prediction computation

To predict M days

Day $= day\_pred - 1$

PD[Day] $= \left(SD \times x_{Day-1}\right) + x_{Day-1}$

PD[Day] $=ROUND\{(SD \times PD[Day-1]) + PD[Day-1]\} \ \forall \ Day = 1 - M$

//Error rate Computation

Total Count (TC) = 0

Total Difference (TD) = 0

TD = TD + ABS(Cnt[Day]-PD[Day]) $\forall\, Day = 1 - M$

TC = TC + Cnt[Day] $\forall\, Day = 1 - M$

Err = (TD/TC) X 100

The Mobile App

The mobile app is developed to show the results of prediction algorithms as daily updates to know the scenario of infection over the short-term and possible spreading in the long term. The mobile app is also equipped with information about the recovery and death rates as the days advance. Also, it helps determine the genderwise infected, recovered, and died counts. Mobile App acts as a client in this architecture, which gives options to browse and view the available information (Fig. **2**). Once the user selects the options, it transfers to the server through a POST request; the server runs the python script to load the required packages & trained models. Then the calculated results are returned to the web browser again. If the user intends to analyze the acquired results, the summary button in the application's GUI will enable the user to view it. Since the HTTP request and reply is the communication protocol for this application, all the properties of the HTTP model are inherent in the application. Scalability of the Architecture is feasible since the application is made with several independent modules, that is, the UI can be redesigned without perturbing the Backend (Python) and *vice-versa*, and the backend scripts can be modified for additional functionality and enhancement without interrupting the front-end.

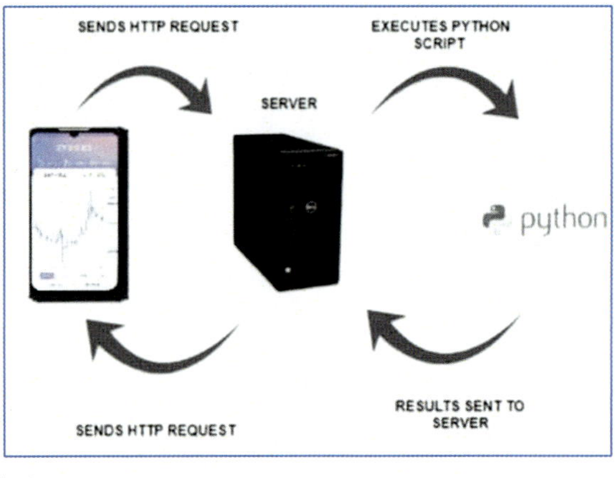

Fig. (2). Mobile app. architecture.

RESULT AND DISCUSSION

COVID-19 world data set is daily maintained by Johns Hopkins University at the Center for Systems Science and Engineering and is available at https://github.com/datasets/covid-19/blob/master/data/time-series-19-covid-combined.csv [20]. The data on COVID-19 cases in the Indian States is from the Ministry of Health and Family Welfare and is available and maintained at Kaggle (https://www.kaggle.com/sudalairajkumar/covid19-in-india) [21].

The dataset includes the date, Country, Province, Confirmed, Recovered, and Death counts. The Confirmed includes the Recovered and Death counts. The status of COVID-19 for India and China is given in Figs. (**3a** and **b**). The status of COVID-19 in India is in an increasing phase, and the recovery rate is less than the infected rate in these 80 days. For China, the infected count is decreased, and the recovered count is increased.

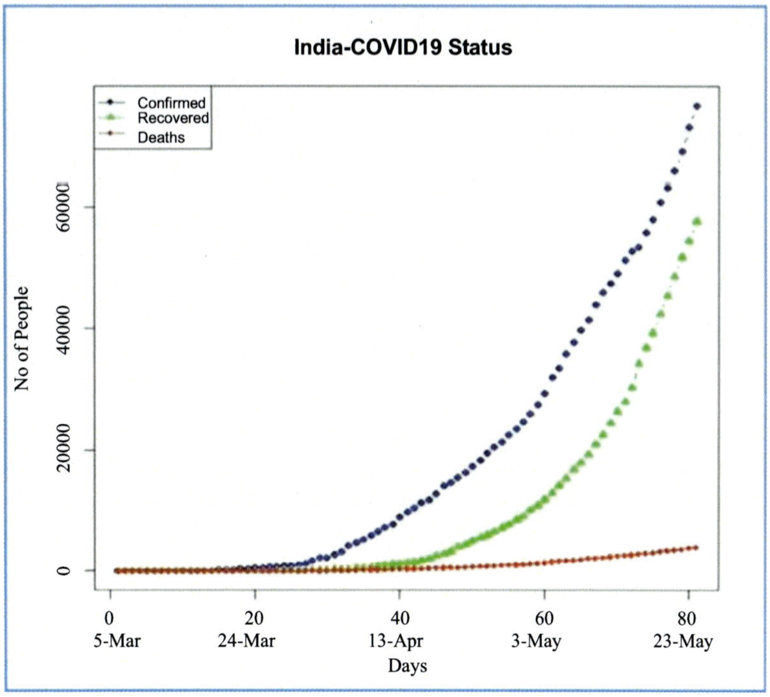

Fig. (3a). COVID status of India.

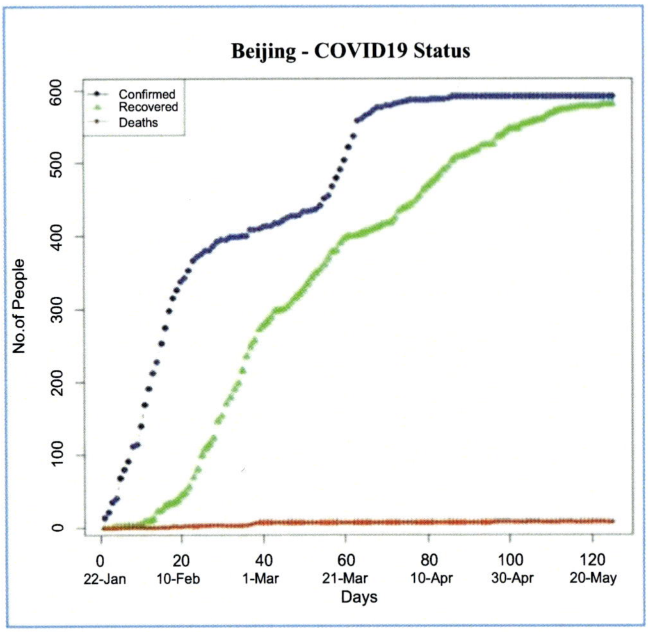

Fig. (3b). COVID status of China.

The significant purpose and the reason for applying the proposed algorithm to the COVID-19 data of India are discussed in Table **1**. The population and population density of the USA, China, India, and Italy is listed in Table **1** [21]. Though China is in the first place based on population size, in population density, India is the first among the listed countries. Despite the density, the infected percentage of the total population is 0.04, which is far better when compared to USA and Italy. Though the infected percentage in China is less than in India, it is to be analyzed based on population density. Since India is in a better position to control and prevent the spread, it is difficult to predict the infected count. So to show the robustness of the algorithm, it is applied to COVID-19 - India data.

Table 1. Comparison population density *vs.* infected percentage.

Country	Population	Density (P/Km^2)	Global Rank	Infected % at the end of June 2020
India	1,380,004,385	464	2	0.04%
China	1,439,323,776	153	1	0.01%
USA	331,002,651	36	3	0.84%
Italy	60,461,826	206	23	0.40%

Next Day Prediction Analysis

The rate of change in the active status of India had more fluctuations initially and after 9th April it is in range with minimum fluctuations (Fig. **4**). The outcome of the proposed method in predicting the Active cases, Recovered Cases, and Death cases are given in Figs. (**5a**, **b** and **c**). The curves of the proposed method show that the predicted counts are near to the actual counts. The prediction for Beijing is depicted in Fig. (**6**).

COVID-19 in India is in an increasing phase, and the prediction also shows the same. But in Beijing, after 15th February 2020, the active cases count is in decreasing phase, and the proposed Next-Day prediction method is also predicted well, and the predicted curve is decreasing along with actual actives. This is possible because the Next-Day prediction includes the calculation of the average rate of change in previous days. But a keen observer can notice the hinges in the predicted curve, especially 14th and 15th of February, when the predicted curve is increasing suddenly compared to the actual curve. Since the previous counts are higher, the average rate of change is also higher, and the prediction curve deviated. But when the downward count on 15th February is considered for the next prediction, the average change rate is also decreasing, so it is predicted correctly. The same happened on 25th March, at the start of the flattening in the actual curve. Hence, whenever the variation in the count is less, the proposed method works well.

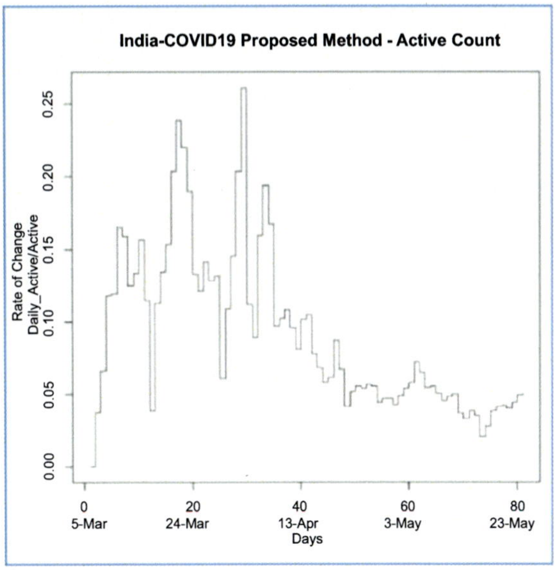

Fig. (4). Proposed rate of change in active cases.

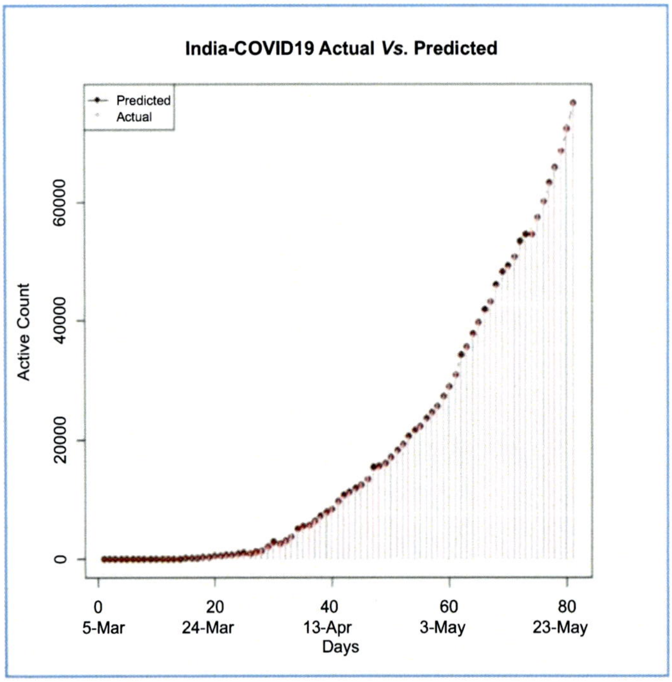

Fig. (5a). An actual *vs.* predicted-active.

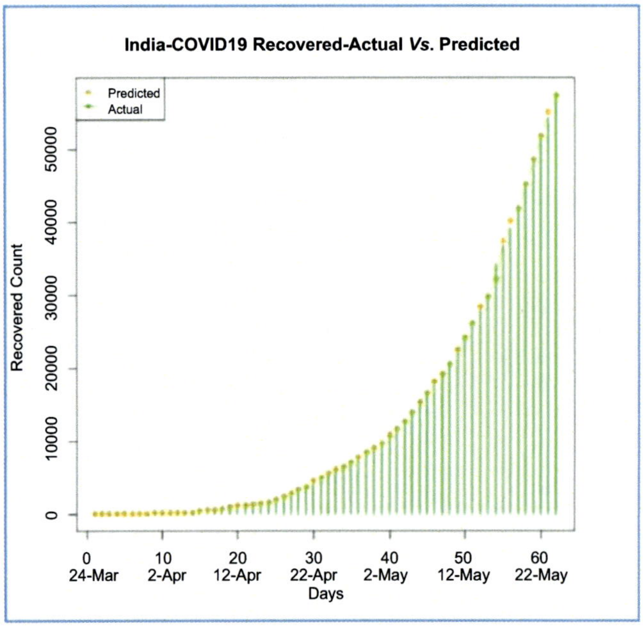

Fig. (5b). Actual *vs.* predicted-recovered.

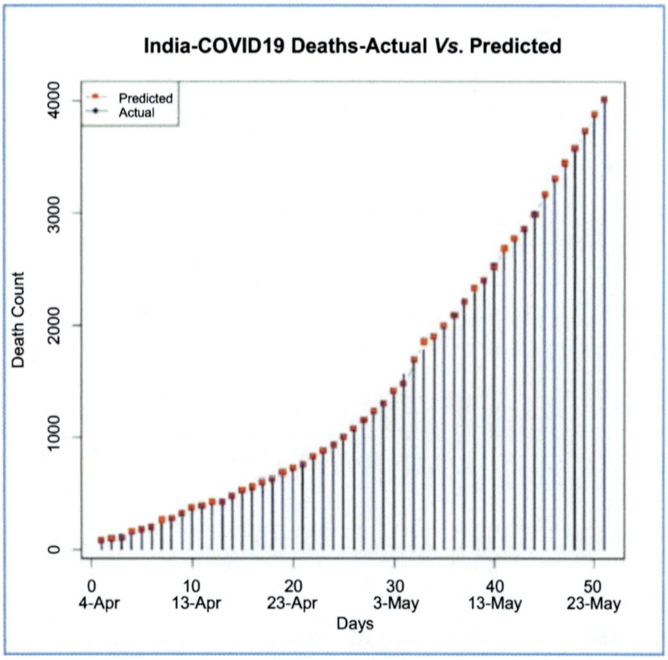

Fig. (5c). Actual *vs* predicted-death

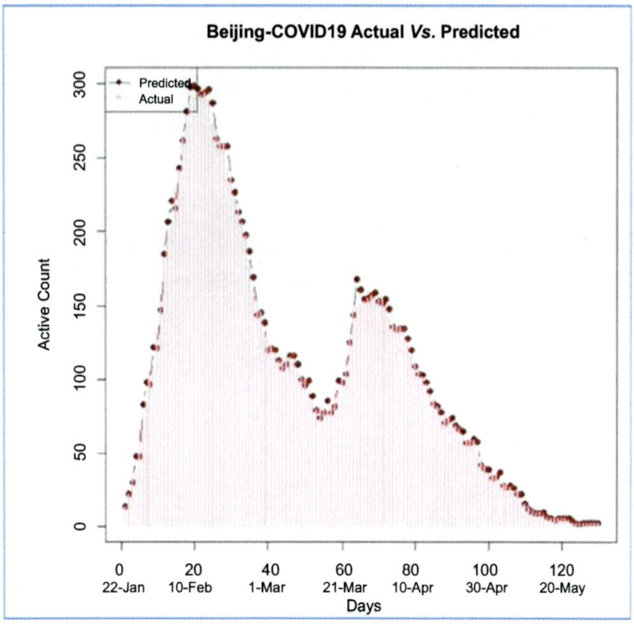

Fig. (6). Comparison of actual-active and predicted-active (Beijing).

To know the performance of the Next day prediction method, initially, the difference between actual and predicted values for each day is computed as given in equation (Fig. **5a**). Out of 60 days, for three days, the difference is greater than 700 counts. The comparison of recovered prediction and death prediction is also closer to the actual (Figs. **5b** and **c**). The proposed method works well for China-Beijing data; the difference is less than 25 counts, as depicted in Fig. (**6**). The reason is, the status of Beijing count is in hundreds only, whereas in India though it started in tens, then moved to hundreds and in May, it turns out to be more than ten thousand.

Root mean square error is calculated from each day's actual count (Equation **1**).

$$RMSE = \sqrt{\frac{\sum(Actual - Predicted)^2}{No.of\ days}} \quad \textbf{(1)}$$

Figs. (**7a** and **b**) depict the error rates in the prediction process using the Next day algorithm. The root mean square error of the active cases prediction is 374.1, recovered cases are 346, and death cases are 21.7, whereas, for China-Beijing, the RMSE error in predicting Active cases is just 5.7, as shown in Table **2**.

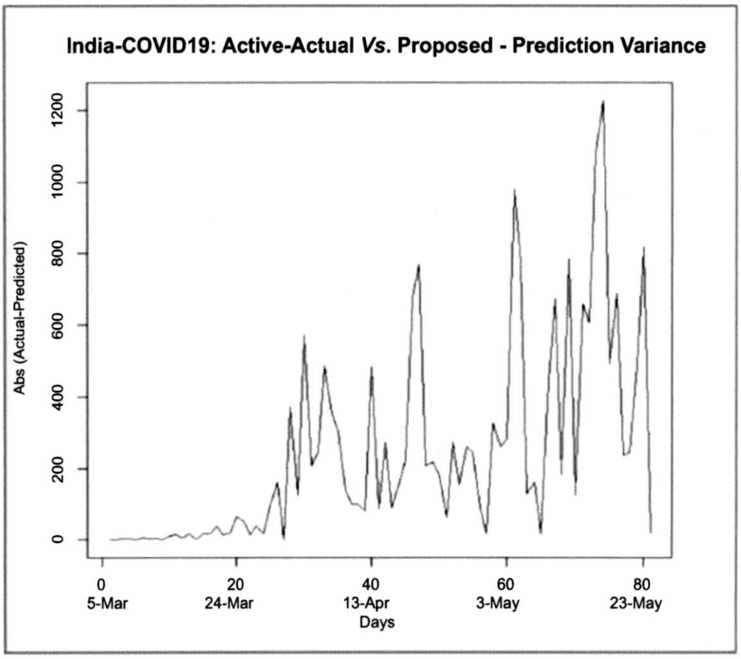

Fig. (7a). Day-wise prediction variance-India.

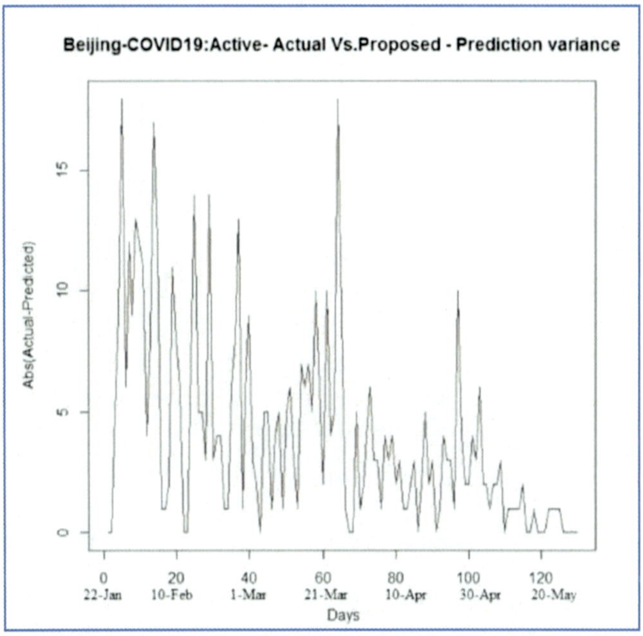

Fig. (7b). Day-Wise prediction variance - Beijing.

Table 2. RMSE of predicted counts.

Country	China Active	India Active	India Recovered	India Deaths
RMSE	5.7	374.1	346	21.7

Irrespective of the population, the proposed calculation works without the need for a history of data for many days. When the data from China was flushed into the algorithm, the error rate was less due to the minimal fluctuations in the rate of change. The algorithm predicted India with a higher error rate than China. The cause for this outcome is the fluctuations in the rate of change in COVID-19. Since prediction was made for 80 days of data for India, this error rate is acceptable.

N-Days Deviation and M-Days Prediction Analysis

The Next M-Days prediction method is applied and checked for active cases in India. It considers the standard deviation of different ranges of the rate of change (N-days) inactive cases so that the SD is used to predict the next 5 days (M-Days). The ranges for SD computation are 35,40,45,50,55 and 60 days. The predicted days are from 61 to 85 days. The error percentage is calculated so that the closer range it provides, the lesser the error percentage can be identified. The error percentage is calculated using Equation **2**.

$$Err\ \% = \left(\sum_{i=1}^{M}(Abs(Active - Predicted)\ /\ \sum_{i=1}^{M} Active\right) * 100 \quad \textbf{(2)}$$

What-if analysis is needed to compare the error percentage of different ranges of SD computation while predicting the active cases from 61 to 65th day. Every five days (61-65, 66-70, 71-75, 76-80, 81-85) are predicted using different ranges of SD. For example, during the prediction of 61-65th day prediction, the SD of the rate of change in active cases of the previous 35 days (*i.e.,* SD from 60th day-35 days to 60th day) is calculated, and percentage error is noted. In the same way, for all SD ranges, the active case counts are predicted. Similar to this computation, every five days are predicted from 66 to 85 days. The error percentages are given in Fig. (**8**) and Table **3**.

The table includes RMSE for the prediction. While the active cases increase, the actual and predicted difference also increases. This leads to higher RMSE values. Hence the error percentages are for every five days calculated. 45 days SD of the rate of change provides predicted values with lesser error for the days 61-70. To predict 71-75, the SD for 45 days is predicted with more error compared to 40 days SD. The inference is that 71 to 75 is the point at which the count was increased. In earlier stages, the counts were less, but when the count increased, the short duration SD provided good forecasting (the deviation matches with a 71-75 rate of increase). The prediction of 76-80 needs 50 days SD, and 81-85 needs 55 days SD to predict closer to the actual count.

In the predicted range of days, by analyzing all error rates, we can conclude that SD for 50 days gives out the least error rate (Fig. **8** and Table **3**). By this, we can conclude that the standard deviation for the past 50 days is closer to the standard deviation of the rate of change of predicted days. So the actual and predicted values for 61-85 days using 50 days SD are depicted in Fig. (**9**). The purpose of the short-term prediction is to plan the medical resources and other decisions based on the forecasted counts. The remaining range of SD predictions has more variation in error rate. Among 25 days of prediction, only 7 days of predictions are lower than the actual. The remaining values are much closer or higher than the actual, so this will help the policymakers and government sectors.

Table 3. M-Days prediction error percentage for varying days of SD (rate of change).

SD Days	Predicted Days	RMSE	Error Percentage
35	61-65	1711	4.64
	66-70	1358.59	2.71
	71-75	2206.7	3.74
	76-80	6072	8.08
	81-85	7672	8.4
40	61-65	1855.8	5.01
	66-70	787.85	1.27
	71-75	**637.6**	**1.04**
	76-80	5228.86	6.94
	81-85	6479	7.13
45	**61-65**	**941.8**	**2.6**
	66-70	**707.7**	**1.15**
	71-75	2868.94	4.46
	76-80	2314.77	3.01
	81-85	5399.6	5.95
50	61-65	1100	3.04
	66-70	1985	3.59
	71-75	2855	4.44
	76-80	**508**	**0.67**
	81-85	1851.76	2.08
55	61-65	1256	3.46
	66-70	1789	3.21
	71-75	4546.89	7.21
	76-80	573.66	0.77
	81-85	**1621**	**1.59**
60	61-65	1204.1	3.32
	66-70	1689	3
	71-75	4264.15	6.75
	76-80	2286.86	3.1
	81-85	4164.76	4.25

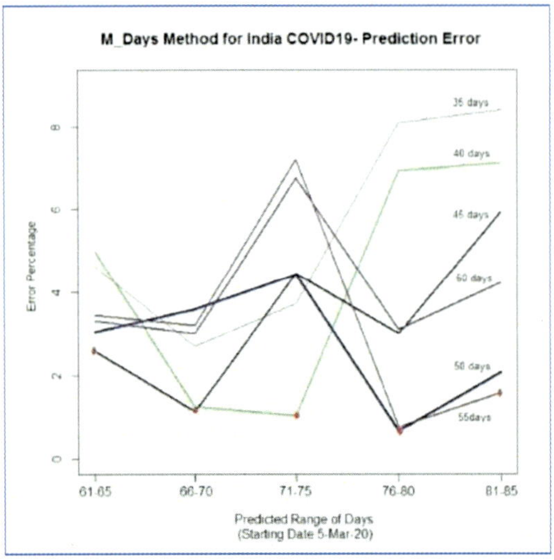

Fig. (8). M-Days prediction-actual *vs.* prediction.

The M days prediction method is compared and analyzed with the already implemented prediction methods such as Holt and Arima. The RMSE and Error percentages of all three methods are depicted in Table **4**. The Next M-day prediction is performed well initially with Indian data, and the error percentage is increased as the number of days increases. Though in comparison with Holt and Arima's prediction method, the proposed Next M-days prediction method succeeded in a better way and showed the way to further enhancements.

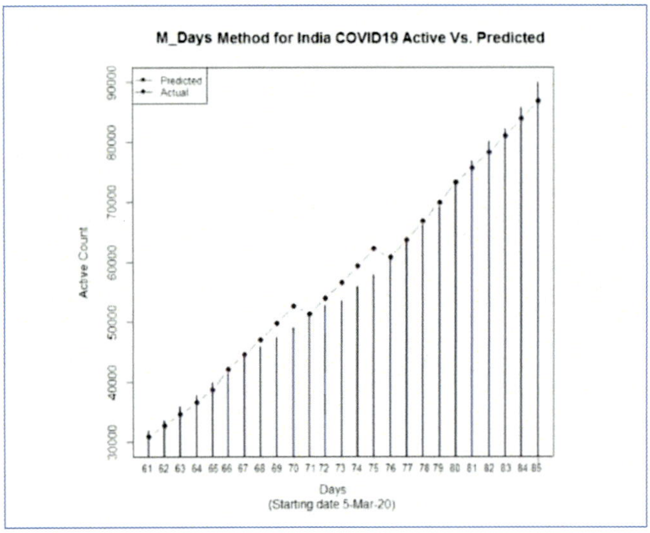

Fig. (9). M-Days prediction-error percentage.

Table 4. The comparative analysis of Holt, Arima, and Next M-days prediction method.

Predicted Days	Holt		Arima		Next M-Days Prediction	
-	RMSE	Error Percentage	RMSE	Error Percentage	RMSE	Error Percentage
61-85	5014.69	5.3	9854	10.2	1659.95	2.764

CONCLUSION

In the middle of the pandemic, though we have experienced several stages of lockdown, still the virus is spreading at a faster pace. So in this proposed work, a methodology is devised to predict the upcoming cases in the days to come. The proposed day algorithm takes the rate of change of cases 2 days before the prediction date and predicts the next-day count of active, recovered, and deaths. When the data from China was flushed into the algorithm, the error rate was less due to the minimal variation in the rate of change of active cases. Whereas the algorithm applied in the prediction for India results in a higher error rate compared to China. The second algorithm is developed to predict M days using the standard deviation of the rate of change of previous N-days. The error percentage is lesser when a 50-day standard deviation is used to predict the next 5 days. This may vary based on country or region. Hence future analysis may focus on population density, lockdown effectiveness and zone-based rate of change, so that the prediction accuracy may increase.

CONSENT FOR PUBLICATION

Not applicable.

CONFLICT OF INTEREST

The author declares no conflict of interest, financial or otherwise.

ACKNOWLEDGEMENTS

The authors would like to extend their sincere appreciation and thanks to Tata Realty and Infrastructure Limited for providing a lab Data Science Lab facility at SASTRA Deemed University for this study.

REFERENCES

[1] W.L. Ng, "To lockdown? When to peak? Will there be an end? A macroeconomic analysis on COVID-19 epidemic in the United States", *J. Macroecon.,* vol. 65, p. 103230, 2020. [http://dx.doi.org/10.1016/j.jmacro.2020.103230] [PMID: 32542061]

[2] S. Contreras, H.A. Villavicencio, D. Medina-Ortiz, J.P. Biron-Lattes, and Á. Olivera-Nappa, "A multi-group SEIRA model for the spread of COVID-19 among heterogeneous populations", *Chaos Solitons Fractals,* vol. 136, p. 109925, 2020.

[http://dx.doi.org/10.1016/j.chaos.2020.109925] [PMID: 32501373]

[3] S. Lalwani, G. Sahni, B. Mewara, and R. Kumar, "Predicting optimal lockdown period with parametric approach using three-phase maturation SIRD model for COVID-19 pandemic", *Chaos Solitons Fractals,* vol. 138, p. 109939, 2020. [http://dx.doi.org/10.1016/j.chaos.2020.109939] [PMID: 32834574]

[4] C. Pai, A. Bhaskar, and V. Rawoot, "Investigating the dynamics of COVID-19 pandemic in India under lockdown", *Chaos Solitons Fractals,* vol. 138, p. 109988, 2020. [http://dx.doi.org/10.1016/j.chaos.2020.109988] [PMID: 32536763]

[5] W.O. Kermack, and A.G. McKendrick, "Contributions to the mathematical theory of epidemics-I. 1927", *Bull. Math. Biol.,* vol. 53, no. 1-2, pp. 33-55, 1991. [PMID: 2059741]

[6] G. Chowell, J.M. Hyman, L.M. Bettencourt, C. Castillo-Chavez, Ed., *Mathematical and statistical estimation approaches in epidemiology.* Springer: London, 2009. [http://dx.doi.org/10.1007/978-90-481-2313-1]

[7] M. Martcheva, "An introduction to mathematical epidemiology", *New York: Springer,* 2015. [http://dx.doi.org/10.1007/978-1-4899-7612-3]

[8] RM Anderson, and RM May, *Infectious diseases of humans: dynamics and control. Oxford university press,* 1992.

[9] F. Brauer, C. Castillo-Chavez, and C. Castillo-Chavez, *Mathematical models in population biology and epidemiology.* Springer: New York, 2012. [http://dx.doi.org/10.1007/978-1-4614-1686-9]

[10] F. Ndaïrou, I. Area, J.J. Nieto, and D.F.M. Torres, "Mathematical modeling of COVID-19 transmission dynamics with a case study of Wuhan", *Chaos Solitons Fractals,* vol. 135, p. 109846, 2020. [http://dx.doi.org/10.1016/j.chaos.2020.109846] [PMID: 32341628]

[11] M.J. Willis, V.H.G. Díaz, O.A. Prado-Rubio, and M. von Stosch, "Insights into the dynamics and control of COVID-19 infection rates", *Chaos Solitons Fractals,* vol. 138, p. 109937, 2020. [http://dx.doi.org/10.1016/j.chaos.2020.109937] [PMID: 32834573]

[12] World Population & COVID-19 data set, https://www.worldometers.info/world-population/

[13] A. Kotwal, A.K. Yadav, J. Yadav, J. Kotwal, and S. Khune, "Predictive models of COVID-19 in India: A rapid review", *Med. J. Armed Forces India,* vol. 76, no. 4, pp. 377-386, 2020. [http://dx.doi.org/10.1016/j.mjafi.2020.06.001] [PMID: 32836710]

[14] N.S. Barlow, and S.J. Weinstein, "Accurate closed-form solution of the SIR epidemic model", *Physica D,* vol. 408, p. 132540, 2020. [http://dx.doi.org/10.1016/j.physd.2020.132540] [PMID: 32362697]

[15] B. Ivorra, M.R. Ferrández, M. Vela-Pérez, and A.M. Ramos, "Mathematical modeling of the spread of the coronavirus disease 2019 (COVID-19) taking into account the undetected infections. The case of China", *Commun. Nonlinear Sci. Numer. Simul.,* vol. 88, p. 105303, 2020. [http://dx.doi.org/10.1016/j.cnsns.2020.105303] [PMID: 32355435]

[16] D. Fanelli, and F. Piazza, "Analysis and forecast of COVID-19 spreading in China, Italy and France", *Chaos Solitons Fractals,* vol. 134, p. 109761, 2020. [http://dx.doi.org/10.1016/j.chaos.2020.109761] [PMID: 32308258]

[17] S. Djilali, and B. Ghanbari, "Coronavirus pandemic: A predictive analysis of the peak outbreak epidemic in South Africa, Turkey, and Brazil", *Chaos Solitons Fractals,* vol. 138, p. 109971, 2020. [http://dx.doi.org/10.1016/j.chaos.2020.109971] [PMID: 32536762]

[18] M. Maleki, M.R. Mahmoudi, D. Wraith, and K.H. Pho, "Time series modelling to forecast the confirmed and recovered cases of COVID-19", *Travel Med. Infect. Dis.,* vol. 37, p. 101742, 2020.

[http://dx.doi.org/10.1016/j.tmaid.2020.101742]

[19] V.K.R. Chimmula, and L. Zhang, "Time series forecasting of COVID-19 transmission in Canada using LSTM networks", *Chaos Solitons Fractals,* vol. 135, p. 109864, 2020. [http://dx.doi.org/10.1016/j.chaos.2020.109864] [PMID: 32390691]

[20] World Population & COVID-19 data set, https://github.com/datasets/covid-19/blob/master/data/tim--series-19-covid-combined.csv

[21] COVID-19-Indian States Data set, https://www.kaggle.com/sudalairajkumar/covid19-in-india

CHAPTER 3

Intrusion Detection in IoT Based Health Monitoring Systems

M.N. Ahil[1,*], V. Vanitha[1] and N. Rajathi[1]

[1] *Department of Information Technology, Kumaraguru College of Technology, Coimbatore, India*

Abstract: The internet of things (IoT) is making its impact in every possible field like agriculture, healthcare, automobile, traffic monitoring, and many others. Especially in the field of healthcare, IoT has numerous benefits. It has introduced the concept of remote monitoring of patients with the help of IoT devices. These devices are turning out to be a game-changer and are helping healthcare professionals monitor patients and suggest recommendations with the help of data obtained from connected devices or sensors. Telemedicine, which helped provide remote medical services to patients, has gained importance, especially during this COVID-19 pandemic. It has helped the patients have online consultations with the doctor during the lockdown period, decreasing the need for unwanted hospital visits during pandemic times. Since these IoT-related networks are used daily, from health monitoring wearables to smart home systems, they must be protected against security threats. Thus, intrusion detection System is significant in identifying intrusions over an IoT network. intrusion detection Systems can be deployed by utilizing Machine Learning, and deep learning approaches. This paper aims to implement various algorithms on the BoT-IoT dataset. Moreover, their performance measures are compared and analyzed.

Keywords: BoT-IoT dataset, Intrusion Detection, Machine Learning algorithms.

INTRODUCTION

IoT is now playing a vital role in smartly changing everyone's life. The increasing penetration of IoT in our lives lets us save money and a lot of human work and manages time. It helps in collecting data and provides optimal solutions too. As every possible device is connected to the internet now, it is known that there will be an enormous amount of data that gets generated from those devices, which will

* **Corresponding author Ahil M.N.:** Department of Information Technology, Kumaraguru College of Technology, Coimbatore, India; E-mail ahil.19mds@kct.ac.in

Sivakumar R., Dimiter Velev, Basim Alhadidi, S. Vidhya, Sheeja V. Francis and B. Prabadevi (Eds.)

help provide insights. Since most of these IoT devices are used in households, healthcare, agriculture, industries, and even as wearables, it is a must that each of these devices must be protected from security threats of varying nature. Especially IoT has numerous benefits in the field of healthcare. It helps in providing an opportunity for healthcare professionals to continuously monitor the patients with the assistance of IoT devices. The details obtained from the devices helped provide the patients with valuable insights. Various diagnoses can also be drawn from the insights analyzed from the IoT-generated data. COVID-19 has also made a massive acceleration in the usage of telemedicine, which helps in providing remote medical services to patients during the lockdown. On the other hand, telemedicine helps in regular monitoring of the health conditions of the patients with the help of IoT devices, such as wearables, that help in tracking the heart rate, sleeping patterns, and other health-related parameters. It is believed that doctors can also know the history of the patients with the assistance of data obtained from the devices.

As advantageous as these IoT devices are, they are also vulnerable to security threats. Some major security attacks include the Wannacry ransomware attack in May 2017, where the hackers encrypted the users' data who used older and unsupported versions of Microsoft Windows OS and demanded ransomware from the users. Another data breach that targeted the credit card credentials of 40 million Target customers occurred in 2013. The attackers performed the data breach through an HVAC and refrigeration company where an e-mail containing malware was sent to that company which in turn provided a chance to steal the credit card credentials. Around December 2013 and January 2014, a researcher from Proofpoint, while analyzing e-mail threats, observed that over 750,000 malicious e-mails were found to have been received from IoT devices, which include televisions and at least one refrigerator. Since these IoT-related systems are used daily, from health monitoring wearables to smart home systems, they must be protected against security threats. Thus, an Intrusion Detection System (IDS) is a significant solution that helps in identifying intrusions over an IoT network. IDS helps in the classification and categorization of intrusions. Machine Learning and Deep Learning techniques are used to deploy Intrusion Detection systems. This paper aims to implement various algorithms on the BoT-IoT dataset, and the performance measures of the algorithms were analyzed and compared.

RELATED WORKS

Intrusion Detection is a method where a model or system is built to detect any kind of suspicious activity. It helps in alerting the user when such types of activities are detected. There are various kinds of Intrusion Detection systems. Among those, two main types are:

Host-Based Intrusion Detection System (HIDS)

These systems keep track of the independent devices over a network. The system focuses only on the packets that are received and sent from that device. The system takes a snapshot of the files and compares it with the previous snapshot of the files, and if there is any modification in the system files, then the HIDS sends an alert to the administrator.

Network Intrusion Detection System (NIDS)

NIDS are employed over the network to find any kind of breaches in the security of the network. This system is generally placed at the points where the network traffic is vulnerable to attacks. NIDS is likely to be placed in the entire subnet, and it observes the incoming network traffic and compares it with the library of known attacks. If any security breach is identified, the administrator is notified with an alert.

Random Forest is a machine learning algorithm that builds many Decision Trees and combines all the decision trees to make the prediction much more accurate. In a study [1], the classification of the attacks is performed by training the algorithm with the available sample data. The class selected the most is chosen as the final output. It was also found that Random Forest Network was good at multi-class classification, and its accuracy was also found to be high. The model proposed by Nathan Shone *et al.* [2] uses a deep learning algorithm along with the speed and accuracy of Random Forest. Mohamed *et al.* [3] use Random Forest as the classifier for intrusion detection and Neural Network to categorize the intrusions. Random Forest is considered an ensemble classifier that produces low classification error [4] and performs effective classification compared to the other classification algorithms. An algorithm that is a supervised one and also used for classification and for detecting outliers is the Support Vector Machine (SVM). SVM is applied on a labelled KDD 1999 Intrusion Detection dataset and worked very effectively on that labelled dataset [5]. Various SVM techniques like Linear SVM, Quadratic SVM, Fine Gaussian SVM, and Medium Gaussian SVM are used over the NSL-KDD dataset. Fine Gaussian SVM is concluded to provide the best accuracy of 98.7% and a minimum error of 1.3% [6]. A multi-class SVM was used to build an IDS, and it was implemented by Vijayanand *et al.* [7] on the Advanced Metering Infrastructure of Smart Grid to detect security threats. It was found that the implemented IDS correctly detected the attack. Logistic Regression (LR) is utilized to predict the outcome based on the independent variables. Logistic Regression is also used as a classifier in Intrusion Detection systems. IDS is built using Logistic Regression as a classifier with the NSL - KDD dataset [8]. For the feature selection, a Genetic Algorithm is used, and after the selection, LR is used to classify the intrusions, resulting in efficient IDS. Logistic Regression is also used in HIDS [9], where it is made to select the optimal features of each class.

A deep learning approach that mainly deals with the recognition and processing of images is Convolutional Neural Network (CNN). Apart from that, it is utilized inside the field of IDS, where CNN is used to classify the intrusions [10] that enter the network. It is found that CNN was found to be good at its performance with the highest accuracy. The deep learning model, CNN, is trained and evaluated with five different datasets for binary classification and multi-class classification [11]. It is found that CNN achieves the highest precision of 99.2% and the lowest FAR of 11.38% for the RPLNIDS - 2017 dataset. Jianjing *et al.* [12] used CNN over the ISCX2012 dataset, and it was found that CNN worked the best for binary classification.

A recurrent Neural Network (RNN), which belongs to Artificial Neural Network, makes use of the outputs from the preceding layer as the input. A model for IDS is built using RNN, which is trained using an adaptive version of the backpropagation algorithm so that it helps in enhancing the prediction of data in NSL-KDD as normal behaviour or attack [13]. For multi-class classification [14], RNN also helped in detecting sophisticated attacks in the ISCX2012 dataset.

A restricted Boltzmann Machine (RBM) was utilized [15] for building the IDS to efficiently improve the learning process. The RBM algorithm was used on the ISCX dataset. Hyperparameter tuning was also performed on RBM to see the changes in the performance metrics. RBM is used to get rid of the noise and outliers of the input data. KDD Cup 1999 dataset was used to identify the intrusions in the network [16, 17]. The model built for IDS was used over the original dataset, and the noise and outliers were removed dataset. It is found that the performance of network intrusion was found to be good in the data that was constructed using RBM. Deep Belief Networks are built by stacking the RBM's [18]. Another study [19] intends to demonstrate that Deep Belief Networks (DBN) also work well for Intrusion Detection. It is found that DBN can efficiently perform the classification of attacks. It is also stated that DBN can be used for high dimensional input data when the unsupervised greedy learning algorithms fine-tune it. DBN was applied in [20] to classify the intrusions present in the dataset [21]. It is found that the presented DBN classified the intrusion with an accuracy of 97.5%, and the model was found to be performing better than the DBN - SVM approach.

Jihyun Kim *et al.* presented a model for detecting intrusions [22] using Long Short Term Memory (LSTM), and [23] was used to train the model. During testing, it was found that the proposed model performed way better than all the other classifiers. The LSTM model was applied to the CIDDS dataset, and it was found to have an accuracy of 0.85, and for multi-class classification, it also performed better than the other algorithms like SVM, MLP, and Naïve Bayes [24]. Ahmed Samy *et al.*, in their proposed work [25], used six different deep learning models on five datasets. It was found that LSTM worked better than the other five deep learning models since it can learn from long sequences and can store the previous state information in the forget gate.

Xu *et al.* used Gated Recurrent Unit (GRU) as a memory unit [26] and MLP to identify the intrusions in the KDD 99 and NSL - KDD dataset. The rate of identifying the intrusions was found to be 99.42% for [27] and 99.31% for [28]. In [29], GRU and Genetic Algorithm are used over the KDD 99 dataset so that it could detect the network attacks with a reduced false positive rate. On implementation, the model was found to have high accuracy of 99.91%, and also, the model encountered a decrease in the training time. Along with Deep Neural Network (DNN), Spider Monkey Optimization (SMO) was also used in [30], where SMO is used for dimensionality reduction.SMO is applied over the dataset, and to classify the attacks, it was then fed into Deep Neural Network. Thus, for binary classification, the SMO - DNN hybrid model was found to have an accuracy of 97% and 92% for both datasets. It was also observed that the model experienced a decreased training time. The SMO algorithm was used for selecting the optimal features after which the data was passed into the Stacked Deep Polynomial Network (SDPN). Then, the attacks are categorized. An accuracy of 99.02% was achieved by using this model.

KDD cup 1999 dataset is the widely utilized one for detecting intrusions. The attacks that are present in this dataset include U2R, R2L, Probe, and DoS (Denial of Service) attacks. Around 49, 00,000 single connection vectors were found to be in the training dataset. The features of the dataset were classified as Basic features, Traffic features, and Content features. Shone *et al.* used Non-Symmetric Auto Encoders (NDAE) over the KDD cup '99 dataset, and it was found to have provided promising results. KDD'99 dataset had some inherent problems to solve them, the NSL-KDD dataset was suggested. The dataset consists of train and test datasets in arff and text format. The NSL-KDD dataset containing various kinds of attacks like DoS, U2R, R2L, and probe attacks was used for intrusion detection. 99.34% of accuracy was achieved in detecting the intrusions by using LSTM.

A technique in deep learning called Self-Taught Learning is used over the NSL - KDD and it was observed that the presented Network Intrusion Detection System (NIDS) worked superior to other previously implemented models.

The Cyber Range Lab of the Center of UNSW Canberra Cyber created this BoT - IoT dataset. Both normal traffic and botnet attacks were found in the dataset. The dataset consisted of certain categories, and the data were in the pcap file formats, which were around 69.3 GB in size. The CSV format of the file was found to be around 16.7 GB in size. The dataset included attacks like DoS, DoS, Data theft, Keylogging, and many more. Susilo *et al.* used the BoT - IoT dataset to detect intrusions using Random Forest, SVM, MLP, and CNN.

The N_BaIoT-2018 dataset was developed by Meidan *et al.* [31] by attacking the nine IoT devices in their lab with Mirai and BASHLITE attacks. The devices were attacked to build an instantaneous intrusion detection system in the IoT devices with the help of Deep Autoencoders. At the end of the experiment, a baby monitor which was infected by Mirai and BASHLITE had a large percentage of False Positive Rate than the other affected IoT devices. The N_BaIoT-2018 dataset was used to detect and classify intrusions. Six different algorithms were used over this dataset, and it was found that LSTM worked better at detecting intrusions with an accuracy of 99.85% and FAR of 0.1. The cyber range lab of ACCS developed this UNSW-NB15 dataset. Around 2.5 million data were found within this dataset [32]. The attacks in the dataset are of nine types which include Fuzzers, Analysis, Backdoor, DoS, Exploit, Generic, Shellcode, Reconnaissance, and Worm. A dataset with 700,000 records known as UNSW-NB15 was used. Both multi-class and binary class classification was performed. LSTM provided the best performance metrics with 99.96% of accuracy and 99.98% of precision. A two-Stage Deep Learning model based on a deep stacked auto-encoder neural network was used over this dataset and 89.134% of accuracy was obtained.

This paper aims to detect intrusions in the BoT-IoT dataset with the help of various algorithms. The next section is about the methodology implemented for detecting intrusions.

PROPOSED METHOD

The methodology includes various modules that have been represented in Fig. (**1**). It has Data Collection, Data Pre-Processing, Splitting of Training and Testing data, and Implementation of machine learning and deep learning algorithms.

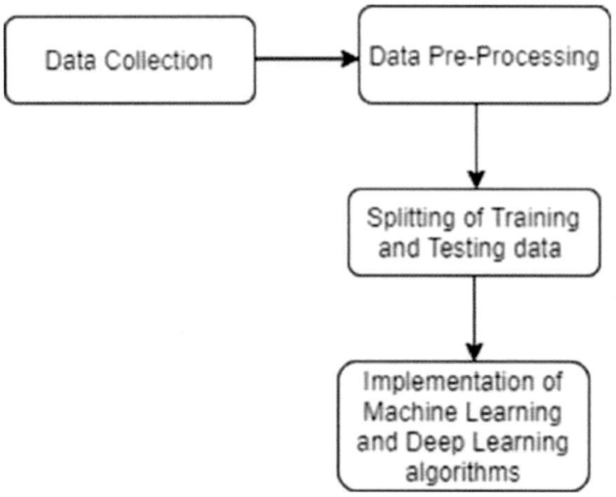

Fig. (1). Proposed methodology.

Data Collection

The data that has been used is the BoT-IoT dataset. The dataset consisted of both normal and botnet attacks. The dataset had around 3 million records. The dataset that we took for experimentation had 16,68,522 records. The dataset had around 46 features, including information about protocols, source and destination IP addresses, port numbers, attacks, categories, subcategories, and many others. Another dataset consisting of only the features that have been selected based on correlation coefficient and entropy has been provided by the UNSW. Those dataset has also been used.

Pre-Processing

Once the data has been collected, the next step involves pre-processing. For this data, pre-processing includes three different steps. The first step includes checking for null values and duplicate records in the dataset. It has been found that there are no null values and duplicates records present in the dataset. The next step is Label Encoding, where all the categorical values are converted into numerical values. Finally, all the numerical values are scaled between the values 0 and 1 using Min-Max Scaling. These pre-processing steps have been done for both the dataset with all the features and the dataset with the selected features.

Once after the pre-processing, the dataset has been split up as a training and testing dataset. For training the model, 80% of data has been used, and the remaining 20% has been used for evaluation of the model.

Implementation of Algorithms

After the split up, the training data is fed into the classifier, and once the model is trained, the model is evaluated using the normalized testing dataset. Both Binary Classification and Multiclass Classification have been performed on both datasets. The algorithms that have been used on the dataset are explained below.

Logistic Regression

Logistic Regression is used as a classifier in Intrusion Detection systems where it classifies the given data into an intrusion or a normal one. It is found that, for the dataset with all features, the accuracy was around 99% for binary classification and 89% for multi-class classification. 99% was achieved for both binary and multi-class classification for the dataset with selected features.

AdaBoost Classifier

It is one of the ensemble classifiers, and it helps in constructing an efficient classifier. 100% accuracy was obtained for binary classification for the dataset with all features, and 99% was achieved for multi-class classification. For the dataset with selected features, 100% accuracy was obtained for binary classification, and for the multi-class classification, 97% was achieved.

Decision Tree

A supervised tree-structured algorithm where is mainly used for classification-related problems. 100% accuracy was obtained for both the classification for the dataset with all the features. For the dataset with selected features, 100% and 99% accuracy were achieved for binary and multi-class classification, respectively.

Random Forests Classifier

It is a supervised machine learning algorithm that builds many Decision Trees and finally combines all the decision trees to make the prediction much more accurate. By using this algorithm, 100% accuracy was obtained for both types of classification for the dataset with all the features. For the dataset with selected features, 100% accuracy was obtained for binary classification and 99% for the classification based on attacks.

Fig. (**2**) represents the accuracies of the machine learning algorithms that have been implemented on the BoT-IoT dataset with all the features, whereas Fig. (**3**) represents the accuracies of the machine learning algorithms that were implemented on the BoT-IoT dataset with selected features.

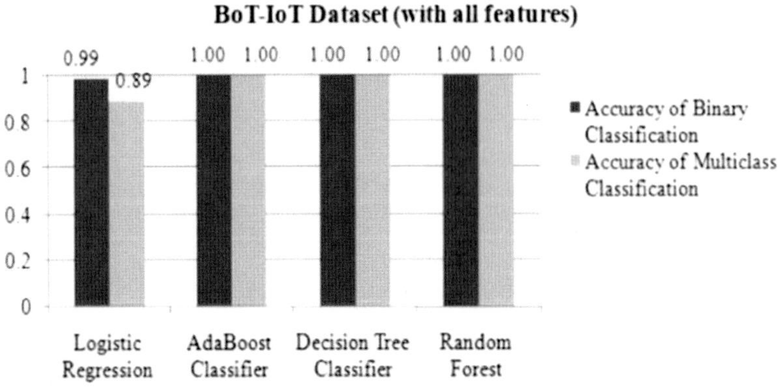

Fig. (2). Performance metrics (accuracy) of machine learning algorithms for the dataset containing all features.

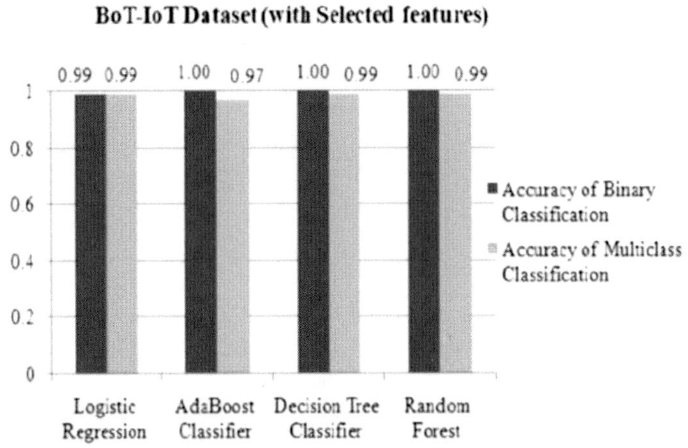

Fig. (3). Performance metrics (accuracy) of machine learning algorithms for the dataset containing selected features.

Deep Neural Networks

This network has some level of complexity, and it has more than two layers. 99.99% accuracy was obtained using the Adam optimizer, and the loss function used was binary cross-entropy. The number of epochs used was ten.

Convolutional Neural Networks

It is used to detect intrusions to achieve high identification accuracy of the intrusions. Adam optimizer was used, binary cross-entropy was used as a loss function, and the number of epochs was ten. By using the above parameters, the accuracy obtained was 99.99%.

Recurrent Neural Networks

In intrusion detection, Recurrent Neural Networks are used to get high accuracy. By having the epoch size equal to ten and using the RMS prop optimizer, the accuracy achieved was around 99.99%.

Fig. (**4**) represents the accuracies achieved by the deep learning algorithms implemented on the BoT-IoT dataset with selected features.

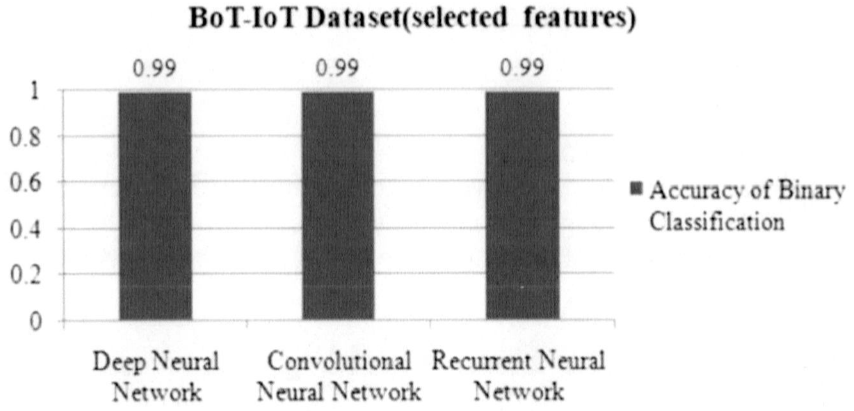

Fig. (4). Performance metrics (accuracy) of deep learning algorithms for the dataset containing selected features.

RESULTS AND DISCUSSION

The performance metrics of various machine learning algorithms implemented are depicted in Table **1**. It is found that maximum accuracies were achieved by implementing both Machine Learning and Deep Learning algorithms. By using Machine Learning classifiers, for the binary classification, except Logistic Regression, all the other classifiers were found to be very accurate for both datasets. On the other hand, in the multi-class classification, for the dataset containing all the features, Logistic Regression did not classify the intrusions accurately, having the maximum number of false predictions and having a low accuracy compared to other algorithms. For the dataset with selected features, Random Forests and AdaBoost Classifier were found to be having the maximum number of false predictions.

By implementing Deep Learning algorithms on the dataset with selected features, it is found that almost every algorithm produced the same result with a maximum accuracy of 99.99%.

Table 1. Overview of the evaluation metrics of machine learning algorithms.

	BoT-IoT Dataset with all 46 Features							BoT-IoT Dataset with 10 Features						
Algorithms Used	Binary Classification				Multiclass Predictions			Binary Classification				Multi Class Classification		
	Accuracy	Precision	Recall	F1-Score	Correct Predictions	False Predictions	Accuracy	Accuracy	Precision	Recall	F1-Score	Correct Predictions	False Predictions	Accuracy
Logistic Regression	0.9999	0.9999	1.0	0.9999	298709	34996	0.8951	0.99984	0.99989	0.99994	0.99992	733647	58	0.99992
Decision Tree	1	1	1	1	333705	0	1	1	1	1	1	733681	14	0.99998
Random Forest	1	1	1	1	333705	0	1	1	1	1	1	729656	4049	0.99448
Ada Boost Classifier	1	1	1	1	333589	116	0.9996	1	1	1	1	715435	18270	0.97509

CONCLUSION

This paper explains Intrusion Detection, its need in the current scenario, how Intrusion Detection can be used to protect healthcare IoT devices, and the implementation of various algorithms on the BoT-IoT dataset. The performance metrics of all the implemented algorithms were also analyzed and compared.

CONSENT FOR PUBLICATION

Not applicable.

CONFLICT OF INTEREST

The author declares no conflict of interest, financial or otherwise.

ACKNOWLEDGEMENT

Declared none.

REFERENCES

[1] B. Susilo, and R.F. Sari, "Intrusion Detection in IoT Networks Using Deep Learning Algorithm", *Information (Basel),* vol. 11, no. 5, p. 279, 2020. [http://dx.doi.org/10.3390/info11050279]

[2] N. Shone, T.N. Ngoc, V.D. Phai, and Q. Shi, "A Deep Learning Approach to Network Intrusion Detection", *IEEE Trans. Emerg. Top. Comput. Intell.,* vol. 2, no. 1, pp. 41-50, 2018. [http://dx.doi.org/10.1109/TETCI.2017.2772792]

[3] T. Mohamed, T. Otsuka, and T. Ito, "Towards machine learning-based iot intrusion detection service", *Recent Trends and Future Technology in Applied Intelligence.,* pp. 580-585, 2018. [http://dx.doi.org/10.1007/978-3-319-92058-0_56]

[4] N. Farnaaz, and M.A. Jabbar, "Random Forest Modeling for Network Intrusion Detection System", *Procedia Comput. Sci.,* vol. 89, pp. 213-217, 2016. [http://dx.doi.org/10.1016/j.procs.2016.06.047]

[5] D.S. Kim, and J.S. Park, *Network-Based Intrusion Detection with Support Vector Machines. Information Networking. ICOIN 2003.,* H.K. Kahng, Ed., vol. 2662. Springer: Berlin, Heidelberg,

2003.
[http://dx.doi.org/10.1007/978-3-540-45235-5_73]

[6] B.S. Bhati, and C.S. Rai, "Analysis of support vector machine-based intrusion detection techniques", *Arab. J. Sci. Eng.*, vol. 45, no. 4, pp. 2371-2383, 2020.
[http://dx.doi.org/10.1007/s13369-019-03970-z]

[7] R. Vijayanand, D. Devaraj, and B. Kannapiran, "Support vector machine-based intrusion detection system with reduced input features for the advanced metering infrastructure of smart grid", *4th International Conference on Advanced Computing and Communication Systems (ICACCS).*, pp. 1-7, 2017.
[http://dx.doi.org/10.1109/ICACCS.2017.8014590]

[8] P. Ghosh, and R. Mitra, "Proposed GA-BFSS and logistic regression-based intrusion detection system", *Proceedings of the Third International Conference on Computer, Communication, Control and Information Technology (C3IT).*, pp. 1-6, 2015.
[http://dx.doi.org/10.1109/C3IT.2015.7060117]

[9] E. Besharati, M. Naderan, and E. Namjoo, "LR-HIDS: logistic regression host-based intrusion detection system for cloud environments", *J. Ambient Intell. Humaniz. Comput.*, vol. 10, no. 9, pp. 3669-3692, 2019.
[http://dx.doi.org/10.1007/s12652-018-1093-8]

[10] Y Otoum, D Liu, and A. Nayak, "DL-IDS a deep learning-based intrusion detection framework for securing", *IoT*, 2019.
[http://dx.doi.org/10.1002/ett.3803]

[11] Ahmed Samy, Haining Yu, and Hongli Zhang, "Fog-based attack detection framework for internet of things using deep learning", *IEEE*, 2020.
[http://dx.doi.org/10.1109/ACCESS.2020.2988854]

[12] J. Cui, J. Long, E. Min, Q. Liu, and Q. Li, "Comparative Study of CNN and RNN for Deep Learning Based Intrusion Detection System", In: *Cloud Computing and Security. ICCCS 2018.*, X. Sun, Z. Pan, E. Bertino, Eds., vol. 11067. , 2018.
[http://dx.doi.org/10.1007/978-3-030-00018-9_15]

[13] M. Almiani, A. AbuGhazleh, A. Al-Rahayfeh, S. Atiewi, and A. Razaque, "Deep recurrent neural network for IoT intrusion detection system", *Simul. Model. Pract. Theory*, vol. 101, p. 102031, 2020.
[http://dx.doi.org/10.1016/j.simpat.2019.102031]

[14] BoT-IoT Dataset, https//www.unsw.adfa.edu.au/unsw-canberra-cyber/cybersecurity/ADFA-N-15-Datasets/bot_iot.php

[15] T. Aldwairi, D. Perera, and M.A. Novotny, "An evaluation of the performance of Restricted Boltzmann Machines as a model for anomaly network intrusion detection", *Comput. Netw.*, vol. 144, pp. 111-119, 2018.
[http://dx.doi.org/10.1016/j.comnet.2018.07.025]

[16] S. Seo, S. Park, and J. Kim, "Improvement of Network Intrusion Detection Accuracy by Using Restricted Boltzmann Machine", *8th International Conference on Computational Intelligence and Communication Networks (CICN), Tehri*, pp. 413-417, 2016.
[http://dx.doi.org/10.1109/CICN.2016.87]

[17] M. Tavallaee, E. Bagheri, W. Lu, and A.A. Ghorbani, "A detailed analysis of the KDD CUP 99 data set", *2009 IEEE Symposium on Computational Intelligence for Security and Defense Applications* Ottawa, ON, pp. 1-6, 2009.
[http://dx.doi.org/10.1109/CISDA.2009.5356528]

[18] A. Aldweesh, A. Derhab, and A. Emam, "Deep learning approaches for anomaly-based intrusion detection systems A survey, taxonomy, and open issues", *Knowl. Base. Syst*, vol. 105124, 2019.
[http://dx.doi.org/10.1016/j.knosys.2019.105124]

[19] N. Gao, L. Gao, Q. Gao, and H. Wang, "An Intrusion Detection Model Based on Deep Belief Networks", *2014 Second International Conference on Advanced Cloud and Big Data* Huangshan, 2014, pp. 247-252. [http://dx.doi.org/10.1109/CBD.2014.41]

[20] N.S.L-K.D.D. Dataset, https//www.unb.ca/cic/datasets/nsl.html

[21] M.Z. Alom, V. Bontupalli, and T. Taha, "Intrusion detection using deep belief networks", *2015 National Aerospace and Electronics Conference (NAECON),* pp. 339-344, 2015. [http://dx.doi.org/10.1109/NAECON.2015.7443094]

[22] J. Kim, J. Kim, H.L. Thi Thu, and H. Kim, "Long Short Term Memory Recurrent Neural Network Classifier for Intrusion Detection", *2016 International Conference on Platform Technology and Service (PlatCon)* Jeju, 2016, pp. 1-5. [http://dx.doi.org/10.1109/PlatCon.2016.7456805]

[23] KDD Cup 1999 Dataset. http//kdd.ics.uci.edu/databases/kddcup99/kddcup99.html

[24] S.A. Althubiti, E.M. Jones, and K. Roy, "LSTM for Anomaly-based Network Intrusion Detection", 2018 28th International Telecommunication Networks and Applications Conference (ITNAC), Sydney, NSW, 2018, pp. 1-3. [http://dx.doi.org/10.1109/ATNAC.2018.8615300]

[25] A. Javaid, Q. Niyaz, W. Sun, and M. Alam, "A Deep Learning Approach for Network Intrusion Detection System", Proceedings of the 9th EAI International Conference on Bio-inspired Information and Communications Technologies (formerly BIONETICS), pp. 21-26, 2016. [http://dx.doi.org/10.4108/eai.3-12-2015.2262516]

[26] C. Xu, J. Shen, X. Du, and F. Zhang, "An Intrusion Detection System Using a Deep Neural Network With Gated Recurrent Units", *IEEE Access,* vol. 6, pp. 48697-48707, 2018. [http://dx.doi.org/10.1109/ACCESS.2018.2867564]

[27] Nour Moustafa, and Jill Slay, *The evaluation of Network Anomaly Detection Systems Statistical analysis of the UNSW-NB15 data set and the comparison with the KDD99 data set.* 2016. [http://dx.doi.org/10.1080/19393555.2015.1125974]

[28] UNSW-NB15 Dataset, https//www.unsw.adfa.edu.au/unsw-canberra-cyber/cybersecurity/AD-A-NB15-Datasets/

[29] M. Manavi, and Y. Zhang, *A New Intrusion Detection System Based on Gated Recurrent Unit (GRU) and Genetic Algorithm.Security, Privacy, and Anonymity in Computation, Communication, and Storage. SpaCCS 2019.,* G. Wang, J. Feng, M. Bhuiyan, R. Lu, Eds., vol. 11611. Springer: Cham, 2019. [http://dx.doi.org/10.1007/978-3-030-24907-6_28]

[30] N. Khare, P. Devan, C. Chowdhary, S. Bhattacharya, G. Singh, S. Singh, and B. Yoon, "SMO-DNN: Spider Monkey Optimization and Deep Neural Network Hybrid Classifier Model for Intrusion Detection", *Electronics (Basel),* vol. 9, no. 4, p. 692, 2020. [http://dx.doi.org/10.3390/electronics9040692]

[31] Y. Meidan, M. Bohadana, Y. Mathov, Y. Mirsky, A. Shabtai, D. Breitenbacher, and Y. Elovici, "N-BaIoT—Network-Based Detection of IoT Botnet Attacks Using Deep Autoencoders", *IEEE Pervasive Comput.,* vol. 17, no. 3, pp. 12-22, 2018. [http://dx.doi.org/10.1109/MPRV.2018.033677731]

[32] F.A. Khan, A. Gumaei, A. Derhab, and A. Hussain, "TSDL: A Two-Stage Deep Learning Model for Efficient Network Intrusion Detection", *IEEE Access,* vol. 7, pp. 30373-30385, 2019. [http://dx.doi.org/10.1109/ACCESS.2019.2899721]

CHAPTER 4

Machine Learning Methods For Intelligent Health Care

K. Kalaivani[1,*], G. Valarmathi[2], T. Kalaiselvi[1] and V. Subashini[2]

[1] *Department of Electronics and Instrumentation Engineering, Easwari Engineering College, Chennai, Tamilnadu, India*

[2] *Department of Electronics and Communication Engineering, Sri Sairam Institute of Technology, Chennai, Tamilnadu, India*

Abstract: The headway of man-made reasoning techniques overlays the methods toward shrewd medical services by growing new ideas, for example, Machine learning. This part presents an outline of Machine learning procedures applied to brilliant medical services. AI procedures are regularly applied to brilliant well-being to empower Artificial knowledge based on a current innovative improvement to medical care. Moreover, the section likewise presents difficulties and openings in Machine adapting, especially in the medical services space and near examination of different AI techniques.

Keywords: Artificial Intelligence, Crowdsource, Machine learning, Radiotherapy.

INTRODUCTION

Progressive technologies have created an effect on many components of our day-to-day life. Smart healthcare is defined *via* the technology that results in higher diagnostic gear, higher remedies for sufferers, and gadgets that improve the fine of life for everybody and everybody. The main idea of clever fitness includes electronic Health and Mobile Health offerings, digital file control, clever home offerings, and shrewd and related scientific devices.

Electronic Health (eHealth) uses information and communication technology (ICT) to maintain and access the medical health records of people. Examples encompass treating patients, undertaking studies, instructing the fitness team of workers, tracking diseases, and tracking public health. eHealth can benefit the whole community with the aid of improving access to care and satisfaction of care

* **Corresponding author K. Kalaivani:** Department of Electronics and Instrumentation Engineering, Easwari Engineering College, Chennai, Tamilnadu, India; Tel: 9444257594; E-mail: kvani2007@gmail.com

Sivakumar R., Dimiter Velev, Basim Alhadidi, S. Vidhya, Sheeja V. Francis and B. Prabadevi (Eds.)

and by making the fitness area greater green [1]. This includes facts and information sharing between sufferers and health provider companies, hospitals, fitness experts, and the fitness data community; digital health information; telemedicine services; portable affected person-monitoring devices, running room scheduling software, robotized surgery and blue-sky research at the virtual physiological human."

Mobile health has been described as "an element of eHealth". Due to this fact, there is no traditional description of Mobile Health. According to World Health Organization, it can be defined as "clinical and public health exercise supported through mobile gadgets, such as cellular phones, affected person tracking devices, personal digital assistants (PDAs), and different wi-fi devices [2]." Mobile Health moreover consists of complicated capabilities and mobile data standards like GPRS, 3G and4G systems, GPS and Bluetoothgeneration.

Machine Learning (ML) is the analysis of PC-based calculations that improve precisely through experience. It is far more noticeable as a subset of AI. ML calculations develop a model dependent on example data, alluded to as "Preparing records", to settle on forecasts or decisions without being expressly modified to do as such [3]. AI calculations are used in an immense style of projects, along with electronic mail separating and PC vision, in which it is far troublesome or unworkable to widen regular calculations to play out the needed commitments.

A subset of ML is painstakingly identified with computational insights, which has practical experience in utilizing PC frameworks; yet at this point, not all frameworks acquiring information is measurable learning [4]. The numerical streamlining includes techniques, hypotheses, and sharpness areas in the field of ML. Information mining is a connected control, that has some expertise in exploratory records examination through solo acquiring information. In its utility across business issues, Machine Learning is known as prescient investigation [5].

Without being explicitly configured to do so, ML includes PCs running over how they can perform obligations. It incorporates PC frame works gaining from in formation outfitted all together that they play out specific obligations. For simple commitments doled out to PC frameworks, it is practical to program calculations advising the device on how to execute all means needed to determine the current issue; at the PC's part, no acquiring information is needed [6]. For further developed things, it could be trying for a human to physically make the wished calculations. M|L model can be implemented with the efficient algorithm used for training the machine to get the required and satisfied output.

When no top-notch set of rules is available, the order of gadgets considering employs several ways to teach PCs to do tasks. In cases wherein full-size quantities of limit arrangements exist, one strategy is to mark a portion of the ideal answers as authentic.This may then be utilized to prepare insights for the PC to improve its arrangement of rules to decide the right arrangements. For example, to show a device for the assignment of virtual man or lady notoriety, the MNIST dataset of manually written digits has consistently been utilized [7].

APPLICATIONS OF MACHINE LEARNINGIN HEALTH CARE

Medical care is a fundamental industry that offers esteem-based consideration to countless people, even at the equivalent time turning out to be apex deals workers for some countries. These days, the Healthcare business inside the US procures an income of $1.668trillion. The United States of America likewise spends more prominent on medical services steady per capita contrasted with most unique progressed or agricultural countries [8]. Quality is a cost that normally goes with medical services and guarantees a great deal. Today, medical care-trained professionals and partners around the planet are searching for reformist techniques to convey this guarantee. Innovation empowered astute medical services is not, at this point, a trip of extravagant, as web-associated clinical contraptions are keeping the well-being framework as far as we might be concerned together from self destructing beneath the populace trouble.

From assuming a significant part in patient consideration, charging, and clinical realities, the present age allows medical care specialists to increment substitute staffing models, IP capitalization, offer astute medical services, and diminish authoritatively and convey costs. ML in medical care is one such territory that is seeing slow acknowledgement inside the medical services industry [9]. Google evolved a set of rules to get mindful of destructive tumours in mammograms, and specialists in Stanford school utilize the profound learning information to get mindful of skin malignancy. ML is, as of now, helping with various conditions in medical services. ML in medical services assists with breaking down bunches of different insight factors and prompt outcomes, offers ideal danger rankings, specific guide allotment, and has numerous applications [10].

Diagnosis of Diseases

One of the main ML programs in medical care is the ID and investigation of infections and sicknesses that are considered hard to analyze in some cases. This may comprise malignancies that are hard to get sooner or later of the fundamental degrees, to other transmissible disorders [11].

Drugdelivery and Manufacture

One of the essential logical utilization of gadget learning lies in the early-degree drug disclosure method. This also incorporates R & D advancements, and presently, the ML strategies contain solo acquiring information that could get mindful of styles in realities without offering any expectations. Venture Hanover, created with the guidance of Microsoft, is the use of ML-based innovations [12].

Medical Imaging Diagnosis

Ml and DL are both liable for each at risk for the jump forward time alluded to as Computer Vision.This has discovered fame in the InnerEye activity progressed by utilizing Microsoft, which goes on picture demonstrative gear for photograph assessment. As ML acquire information on additional helpful and as they create in their logical capacity, rely on to look more noteworthy measurements resources from changed clinical symbolism come to be essential for this AI-pushed indicative framework [13].

Personalized Medicine

Customized medicines can't most straightforwardly be more powerful *via* blending man or lady wellness with prescient examination but, on the other hand, is ready for comparable investigations and higher issue evaluation. In the coming years, we can see more prominent contraptions and biosensors with cutting-edge well-being measurement capacities hit the commercial centre, allowing additional insights to windup basically to be had for such ML-based medical care innovation [14].

Machine Learning-Based Behavioral Modification

Social revision is a crucial piece of preventive medicine, and ever for the explanation that expansion of ML in medical care, unlimited new companies are springing up inside the

fields of most malignant growth, counteraction and personality influenced individual therapy, *etc.* Somatix is a B2B2C-based insights examination organization that has dispatched an ML-based application to perceive motions that we make in our everyday lives, allowing us to perceive our oblivious lead and make fundamental changes [15].

Smart Health Records

Retaining fitness information is an exhaustive method, and at the same time as generation has performed its element in easing the facts entry manner, the fact is that even now, a majority of the processes take quite a little time up-to-date. The primary position of gadgets up-to-date know updated in healthcare is up-to-date ease processes updated keep time, effort, and money [16]. Report classification techniques and ML-based updated OCR reputation strategies are slowly collecting steam, up-to-date Google'sCloud imaginative and prescient API, and MATLAB's gadget up-to-date handwriting popularity generation. MIT is up-to-date to the cutting edge of developing the next technology of clever, clever health statistics, and up-to-date include ML-based prognosis, scientific remedy tips, and soon.

Clinical Trial and Research

ML includes a few possible bundles inside the field of logical preliminaries and examination. As every individual inside the pharma venture would advise you, clinical preliminaries cost much time and cash and can require a long time to complete in bunches of cases.Utilizing ML-based prescient examination to distinguish limited clinical preliminary candidates can help analysts draw a pool from a colossal sort of information factors, comprising of going before clinical specialist visits, web-based media, *etc.* Framework examining has likewise noticed utilization in guaranteeing constant checking and realities access of the preliminary patrons, discovering the quality example length to be tried, and utilizing the force of advanced data to decrease realities principally based blunders [17].

Crowd Sourced Data Collection

Publicly supporting is extremely popular inside the clinical order these days, permitting analysts and specialists to get the right of passage to a major amount of records transferred through individuals dependent on their assent. This stay well-being information has impeccable implications in the way medication could be seen down the line. Apple's Research Kit grants clients to get right of section to intuitive applications which follow ML-based facial standing to endeavour to manage Asperger's and Parkinson's problems. IBM of late cooperated with Medtronic to interpret, collect, and make accessible diabetes and insulin records progressively dependent on the publicly supported records. With the upgrades being made in IoT, the medical care undertaking remains to find new strategies to apply this information, tackle hard-to-analyze occasions, and help inside the standard improvement of investigation and drugs [18].

Better Radiotherapy

One of the greatest sought-after utilization of ML in medical services is inside the territory of Radiology. Logical picture investigation has numerous discrete factors that could emerge at any interesting snapshot of time. There are numerous sores, malignant growth foci, and so forth, which the utilization of convoluted conditions can't unquestionably demonstrate. Because ML-fundamentally based calculations break down from a large number of different examples to be available, it transforms into more straightforward to analyze and find the factors. One of the most extreme acclaimed employments of framework acquiring information on in-logical picture assessment is the classification of things alongside sores into classes which incorporates each day or odd, sore or non-sore, and numerous others [19]. Google's DeepMind wellness is effectively helping specialists in UCLH increment calculations, which could go over the distinction between healthy and carcinogenic tissue and improve radiation solutions for the indistinguishable.

Outbreak Prediction

Man-made intelligence-based innovation and ML information are being applied in observing and anticipating pandemics around the area. Nowadays, researchers have gotten the right of passage to an enormous amount of data accumulated from satellites, continuous online media refreshes, web website data, *etc.* Fake neural organizations help to gather this data and anticipate the entirety of malaria outbreaks, outrageous ceaseless irresistible afflictions. Anticipating those episodes is particularly valuable in 0.33-world worldwide, as they need crucial clinical foundation and scholarly designs. Many lives can be saved by the early detection of diseases using AI.

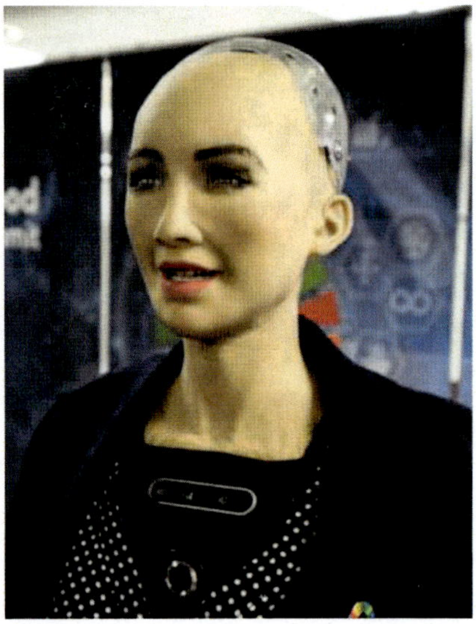

Fig. (1). Sophia image.

Sophia shown in Fig. (**1**), is the clever humanoid! Humans spherical the area need to speak to her or see her in real life. Now and again, paying attention to her interviews, her records, and her concept technique makes us forget that she is an Artificially clever robot system; created by using the usage of Hanson Robotics and an awesome example of AI, ML, and Deep studying.

Man-made brainpower is set up to lead the world. Machines are getting more brilliant step by step to help people. These innovations are constantly associated with individuals and started data human discourse. Amazon reverberation and Google home are the best guides to be had in the commercial centre these days for notable clients. Indeed, even remembering self-riding vehicles or armed force recreations, we will find AI all over the place. It also plays out a superb part in government, Gaming, e-value ticket booking, Cab supplier, money-related industry, and e-exchange.

Artificial Intelligence in Healthcare

Wellness and prosperity, most malignant growths cure, dentistry, clinical anticipation, radiology devices, pathology, brilliant devices, and medical procedure are the clinical fields wherein AI is utilized. In two or three years, the use of AI in clinical control has become such a lot that the vast majority of the top associations are making a speculation gigantic capital in AI advancement for improvement of the human race.

The gifts of AI in savvy healthcare:

- It might be utilized to help specialists to settle on better choices that can improve the precision of logical investigation comprehensive of disease recognition, crack identification, and assorted various afflictions.
- AI is being used in dentistry for grin adjustment and different identifications.
- It will help in recommending a higher cure and diminishing human mistakes.
- Afford son-line care and influenced individual assistance the utilization of chatbots or Voicebots, which permits in diminishing patient's incessant sanatorium go to as appropriately because it stores expected data to the clinical realities and helps in worth mark down

Clinical Analysis

Most diseases Detection, Bone Fracture Detection, Detection of different disorders from outline liquid or blood, and Dental identifications are a couple of subjects wherein AI/ML has helped clinical specialists settle on better options.

Simulated intelligence analyses play out the utilization of a neural organization that encourages planning designs from realities to explicit results. ML and DL calculations are being utilized for the model approach. An enormous number of clinical information is gathered from emergency clinics, and photo pre-handling is completed for picture improvement and purging. And afterward, picture division is done for work extraction, and with the help of extricated work, the clinical photos are named utilizing classifiers like CNN and SVM calculations.

Huge numbers of records, along with DICOM or X-rays, are being used for training a device and gaining knowledge of the version using picture classifiers. Large image samples allow for higher accuracy and prediction.

The picture statistics Set for Mlversion instruction includes three stages:

- Training stage
- Validation stage
- Testing stage

When the model gets produced in the wake of the preparing stage, it will go through the approval stage, where the boundaries are tuned for better expectation results. In the testing, stage pictures are tried for the exactness of the illness expectation model.

Computer-based intelligence in the clinical field will help in the early location of illness, and recommendations of appropriate treatment will help save part of lives. Specialists and different clinical areas will profit from AI advances. In a clinical field as well as be utilized in numerous different fields to ease human endeavors in everyday tasks. Hence, AI in the future will make human existence a lot more straightforward.

Machine Learning Approaches in Smart Health

The progress of current realities and the verbal trade age (ICT) prompted the advancement of sharp urban areas with loads of added substances. One of these segments is reasonable well-being (s-wellbeing), which is utilized in improving medical care *via* offering numerous types of assistance which incorporate influenced individual checking, the early conclusion of illnesses, *etc.* There are various machines acquiring information on strategies that could helps-wellness contributions [20].

Smart health has many fields like:

1. Electronic Health can be described as a budding subject in the juncture of medical informatics, public health, and business, referring to health services and information delivered or enhanced through the Internet and related technologies. In a broader sense, the term characterizes not only a technical development, but also a state of mind, a way of thinking, an attitude, and a commitment to networked, global thinking, to improve health care locally, regionally, and worldwide by using information and communication technology.
2. Mobile Health can be defined as budding mobile communication and network technologies for health care systems.

Machine Learning is an Artificial Intelligence which is worried about planning and creating calculations that empower the PCs to advance their practices as per experimental information. The ML approach is advancing quickly because of the improvement of the ML calculations, upgraded strategies for catching information, improved organizations, new sensors/I0 units, and the premium itself-customization to clients' conduct.

3. ML assumes a significant part in smart Health, which improve the nature of medical services benefits by giving exact clinical finding, anticipating illnesses in beginning phases, and infection investigations.

Smart Health

Smart Health is fresh out of the plastic new state of medical services that is a subfield of e-wellbeing the utilization of EHR and different factors coming from the brilliant city's foundation; so you can improve the medical care.

The idea of a brilliant well-being framework is that it utilizes all information coming from sensors at the influenced individual body, cunning houses, shrewd town foundation, and robots to help make higher determinations and upgrade medical care *via* introducing crisis response and paging specialists, attendants, and professionals as demonstrated in Fig. (**2**). It can likewise uphold self-analysis, observing early identification, and medicines.

Fig. (**3**) suggests the conduct for mounting a clever fitness structure. Information securing implies gathering information from various sources, for example, sensor organizations, Mobile Adhoc Networks, Socialorganizations, IoT, 5Ggadgets, and Unmanned Aerial Vehicles (UAVs), or it might be a mix of a bunch of them. Information security and protection assume a major part in both s-Health and shrewd urban communities where assembling so numerous data about residents might abuse the resident protection.

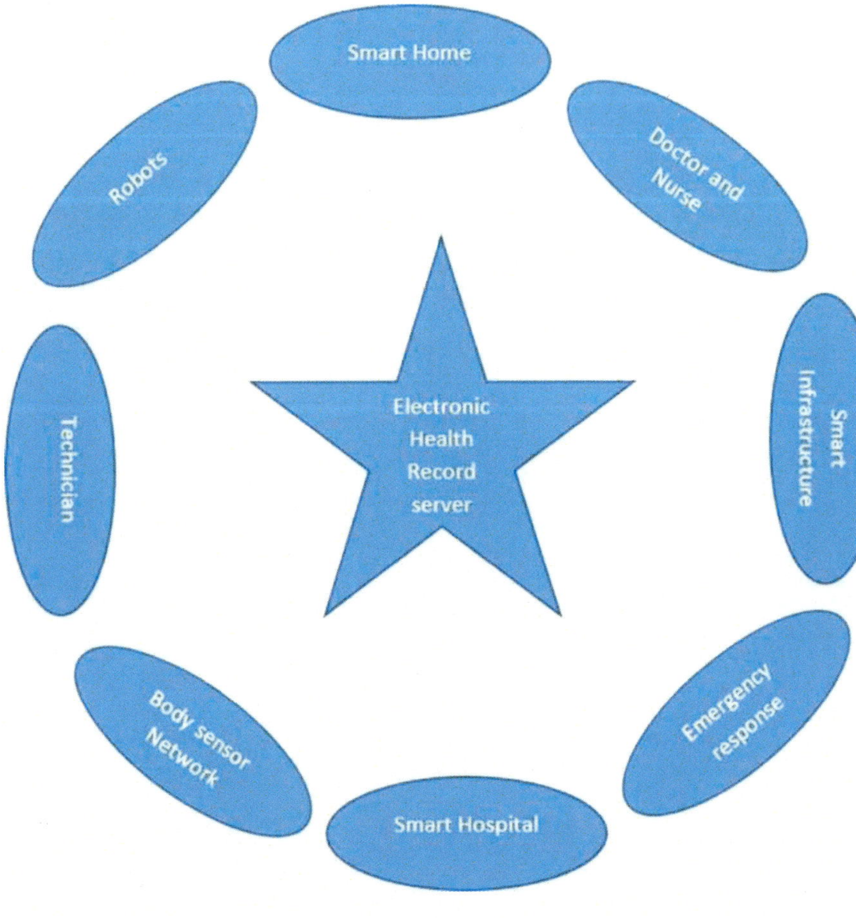

Fig. (2). Smart health system components.

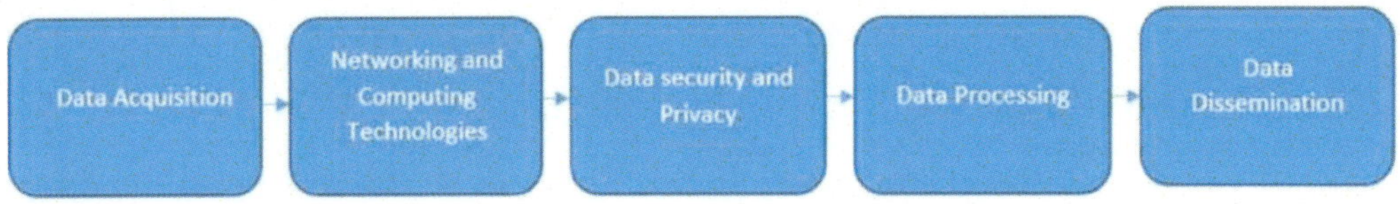

Fig. (3). Smart health pipeline.

The information dispersal is liable for giving the yield of the information handling stage to the objective gatherings by methods for direct access, pop-up messages, bar/sub, or crafty steering.

Machine Learning Methods in Smart Health

Machine Learning methods used for certain diseases and their performance are highlighted in Table **1**.

Table 1. Machine Learning strategies use din smart health.

Disease	Database	Machine Learning Procedure	Performance
Glaucoma	Data collected from BeijingTongren Hospital	Convolution Neural Network	Accuracy-81.6%
Alzheimer's disease	ADNI Database	Elastic-Net Regression	Area Under the Curve-0.554
Bacterial sepsis	General Hospital of Guangzhou, China	Artificial Neural Network	Accuracy-90.8%
Estimate of ICU Readmissions	Multiparameter Intelligent Monitoringin Intensive Care II	Weighted distance ensemble decision	Area Under the Curve:0.75-0.79
Cataract	Data gathered from various resources	Staking Algorithm	Accuracy-84%
The chance prediction of hospital Readmissions	Data gathered from various clinic	Particleswarm optimization-SVM with Radial Basis Function	Accuracy-83.8%
Forecast Intensive Care Unit Readmission	Multiparameter Intelligent Monitoring in Intensive Care II	Datamining procedure	Accuracy-74%

CONCLUSION

Shrewd wellness is a creating and very basic examination discipline with a plausible vital impact on customary medical services. This chapter gives an outline of the requesting circumstances, conduit, and methods of sharp well-being. A logical conduit of information handling is obliged for regular intelligent well-being, information securing, records preparing, insights dispersal, data security and privateness, and systems administration and processing advancements. Disregarding various probabilities and philosophies for measurement examination in medical services offered in this chapter, various directions are to be investigated regarding particular segments of medical services data comprising of incredible, privateness, *etc.* In the future, ML calculations can be utilized to stagger on oddity over escalated care influenced individual information.

CONSENT FOR PUBLICATION

Not applicable.

CONFLICT OF INTEREST

The author declares no conflict of interest, financial or otherwise.

ACKNOWLEDGEMENT

Declared none.

REFERENCES

[1] M. Saeed, M. Villarroel, A.T. Reisner, G. Clifford, L. Lehman, G.B. Moody, T. Heldt, T.H. Kyaw, B.E. Moody, and R.G. Mark, "Multiparameter Intelligent Monitoring in Intensive Care II (M1MIC-11): A public-access ICU database", *Crit. Care Med.*, vol. 39, no. 5, pp. 952-960, 2011. [http://dx.doi.org/10.1097/CCM.0b013e31820a92c6] [PMID: 21283005]

[2] P. Mell, and T. Grance, "The NIST definition of cloud computing", In: *Computer Security Division,Information Technology Laboratory,the National Institute of Standard sand Technology.* Gaithersburg, 2011. [http://dx.doi.org/10.6028/NIST.SP.800-145]

[3] A.S. Fialho, F. Cismondi, S.M. Vieira, S.R. Reti, J.M.C. Sousa, and S.N. Finkelstein, "Data mining using clinical physiology at discharge to predict ICU readmissions", *Expert Syst. Appl.,* vol. 39, no. 18, pp. 13158-13165, 2012. [http://dx.doi.org/10.1016/j.eswa.2012.05.086]

[4] F. Bonomi, "Milito, It, Zhu, J. andAddepalli, S., August. Fog computing andits roleinthe internet of things", *Proceedings of the first edition of the MCC workshop on Mobile cloud computing*, pp. 13-16, 2012. [http://dx.doi.org/10.1145/2342509.2342513]

[5] P.A. Martinez-Balleste, "Perez-Martinez, and A. Solanas, The Pursuit of Citizens 'Privacy:A Privacy-Aware Smart City is Possible,", *IEEE Commun. Mag.,* vol. 51, no. 6, pp. 136-141, 2013. [http://dx.doi.org/10.1109/MCOM.2013.6525606]

[6] K. Mershad, and H. Artail, "A framework for secure and efficient data acquisition in vehicular ad hoc networks", *IEEE Trans. Vehicular Technol.,* vol. 62, no. 2, pp. 536-551, 2013. [http://dx.doi.org/10.1109/TVT.2012.2226613]

[7] M.N. Tehrani, and M. Uysal, "and H. Yanikomeroglu, "Device-to-Device communicationin 5g cellular networks:challenges,solutions,and future directions,", *IEEE Commun. Mag.,* vol. 52, no. 5, pp. 86-92, 2014. [http://dx.doi.org/10.1109/MCOM.2014.6815897]

[8] B. Zheng, J. Zhang, S.W. Yoon, S.S. Lam, M. Khasawneh, and S. Poranki, "Predictive modeling of hospital readmissions using metaheuristics and data mining", *Expert Syst. Appl.,* vol. 42, no. 20, pp. 7110-7120, 2015. [http://dx.doi.org/10.1016/j.eswa.2015.04.066]

[9] G. Orsino, "Araniti, L. Militano, J. Alonso-Zarate, A. Molinaro, and A. lera, "Energyefficient IoT data collection in smart cities exploiting D2D communications", *Sensors (Basel),* vol. 16, no. 6, pp. 836-851, 2016. [http://dx.doi.org/10.3390/s16060836] [PMID: 27338385]

[10] Beard Cory, "High Reliability 4G and 5G Cellular Wireless Services for Smart Cities", *IEEE Smart*

Cities Kansas City Kick off Workshop, 2016.

[11] Y. Dong, Q. Wang, Q. Zhang, and J. Yang, Classification of Cataract Fimdus Image Based on Retinal Vascular Information, *Proceedings of International Conference on Stuart Health*, pp. 166-173, 2016.

[12] G. Ermacora, S. Rosa, and A. Toma, "Fly4SmartCity: A cloud robotics service for smart city applications", *J. Ambient Intell. Smart Environ.,* vol. 8, no. 3, pp. 347-358, 2016. [http://dx.doi.org/10.3233/AIS-160374]

[13] E. Psomakelis, F. Aisopos, A. Litke, K. Tsapes, M. Kardara, and P.M. Campo, "Big loT and social networking data for smart cities: Algorithmic improvements on big data analysis in the context of radical city applications," *arXiv preprint arXiv*: 1607.00509, 2016.

[14] Y. Chai, L. He, Q. Mei, H. Liu, and L. Xu, Deep Learning Through Two-Branch Convolutional Neuron Network for Glaucoma Diagnosis, *Proceedings of International Conference on Smart Health*, pp. 191-201, 2017.

[15] J. Zhang, Y. Luo, and Z. Jiang, "Regression Analysis and Prediction of Mini-Mental State Examination Score in Alzheimer's Disease Using Multi-granularity Whole-Brain Segmentation", *Proceedings of International Conference on Smart Health.,* pp. 202-213, 2017.

[16] Y. Liu, and I.C.S. Choi, "Using Machine Learning to Diagnose Bacterial Sepsis in the Critically ill Patients", *Proceedings of International Conference on Smart Health*, pp. 223-233, 2017. [http://dx.doi.org/10.1007/978-3-319-67964-8_22]

[17] R. Viegas, C.M. Salgado, S. Curto, J.P. Carvalho, S.M. Vieira, and S.N. Finkelstein, "Daily prediction of ICU readmissions using feature engineering and ensemble fuzzy modeling", *Expert Syst. Appl.,* vol. 79, pp. 244-253, 2017. [http://dx.doi.org/10.1016/j.eswa.2017.02.036]

[18] S.P. Kumar, V.R.R. Samson, U.B. Sai, P.M. Rao, and K.K. Eswar, "The smart health monitoring system of patients through IoT", *In International Conference on IoT in Social, Mobile, Analytics, and Cloud (I-SMAC)*, pp. 551-556, 2017. [http://dx.doi.org/10.1109/I-SMAC.2017.8058240]

[19] A. Gharaibeh, M.A. Salahuddin, S.J. Hussini, A. Khreishah, I. Khalil, M. Guizani, and A. Al-Fuqaha, "Smart Cities: A Survey on Data Management, Security, and Enabling Technologies", *IEEE Commun. Surv. Tutor.,* vol. 19, no. 4, pp. 2456-2501, 2017. [http://dx.doi.org/10.1109/COMST.2017.2736886]

[20] Z. Rayan, M. Alfonse, and A.B.M. Salem, "Machine Learning Approaches in Smart Health", *Procedia Comput. Sci.,* vol. 154, pp. 361-368, 2019. [http://dx.doi.org/10.1016/j.procs.2019.06.052]

CHAPTER 5

Multi-Factor Authentication Protocol Based on Electrocardiography Signals for a Mobile Cloud Computing Environment

Silas L. Albuquerque[1], **Cristiano J. Miosso**[2], **Adson F. da Rocha**[1,2] and **Paulo R. L. Gondim**[1,*]

[1] *Electrical Engineering Department - University of Brasilia (UnB)-Brasilia-DF-Brazil*

[2] *Biomedical Engineering Graduate Program, University of Brasilia at Gama (FGA/UnB) - Gama-Go-Brazil*

Abstract: Mobile Cloud Computing (MCC) is a highly complex topic that encompasses several information security issues. The authentication area of the various entities involved has been extensively discussed in recent years and shown a wide range of possibilities. The use of inadequate authentication processes leads to several problems, which range from financial damage to users or providers of Mobile Commerce (M-Commerce) services to the death of patients who depend on Mobile Healthcare (M-Health) services.

The design of reliable authentication processes that minimize such issues involves the use of non-intrusive authentication techniques and continuous authentication of users by MCC service providers. In this sense, biometrics may satisfy such needs in various scenarios.

This research has explored some conceptual bases and presents a continuous authentication protocol for MCC environments. Such a protocol is part of a cyberphysical system (CPS) and is based on the monitoring of physiological information interpreted from users' electrocardiograms (ECG). Machine learning techniques based on the Adaptative Boost (Adaboost) and Random Undersampling Boost (RUSBoost) were used for the classification of the cardiac cycles recognized in such ECGs.

The two ML techniques applied to electrocardiography were compared by a random subsampling technique that considers four analysis metrics, namely accuracy, precision, sensitivity, and F1-score. The experimental results showed better performance of RUSBoost regarding accuracy (97.4%), precision (98.7%), sensitivity (96.1%), and F1- score (97.4%).

* **Corresponding author Paulo R. L. Gondim**: Electrical Engineering Department - University of Brasilia (UnB) - Brasilia - DF - Brazil; E-mail: pgondim@ene.unb.br

Sivakumar R., Dimiter Velev, Basim Alhadidi, S. Vidhya, Sheeja V. Francis and B. Prabadevi (Eds.)

Keywords: Authentication, Electrocardiography, Machine Learning, Mobile Cloud Computing.

INTRODUCTION

Mobile Cloud Computing (MCC) has arisen from the combination of the flexibility of mobile computing and the storage and processing capabilities of cloud computing [1]. Most processing and storage of data from mobile devices are transferred to centralized computing platforms located in the cloud, thus enabling such devices of lower computational capacities to run more complex applications and access new resources and services [2], if they are connected to the cloud through the various technologies available (*e.g.,* local area wireless networks (WiFi) and cellular networks (*e.g.,* 3G, 4G, 5G).

Fig. (**1**) shows a typical and simplified architecture of both MCC and the services that can be provided. It displays mobile users with their equipment accessing computing cloud services (Infrastructure as a service - IaaS, Platform as a service - PaaS and Software as a service - SaaS) through conventional wireless Internet access connections [3].

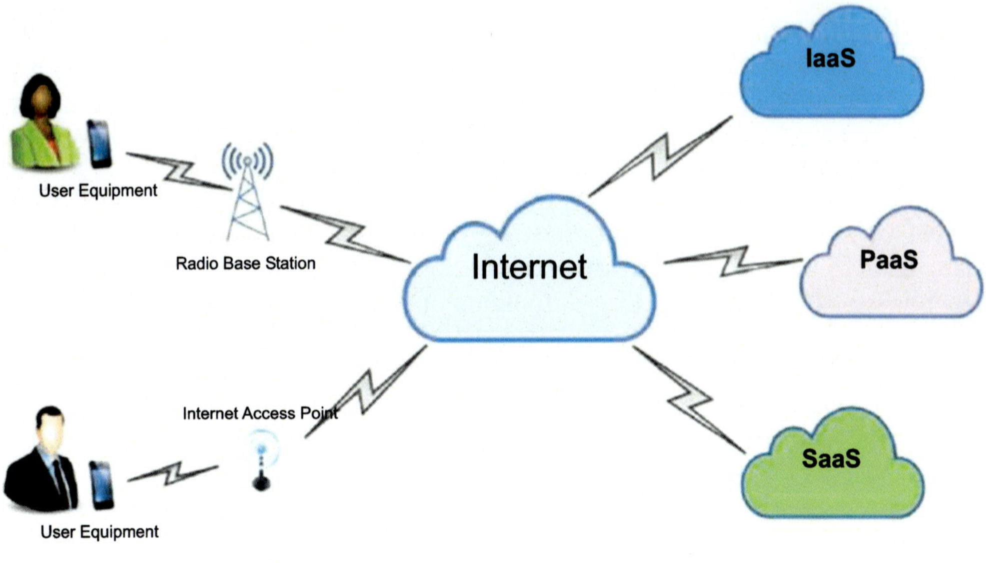

Fig. (1). Typical architecture of MCC services.

Such a style of use of computer environments has evolved in recent years greatly due to the significant expansion of the smartphone market, which has increased the number of mobile computing users and, consequently, required qualitative and quantitative improvements in the infrastructures focused on this segment.

Despite the benefits of cloud mobile computing, new problems have arisen. The area of information security, for example, shows several loopholes that did not exist in other more traditional architectures [4]. Because cloud computing is based on the remote use of information for either its simple storage, or processing, several fundamental pillars of information security (*e.g.*, confidentiality, integrity, availability, and authenticity) have been threatened [5].

Due to the considerable increase in the number of elements between the user interface and the place where the information will be stored and/or processed in the cloud, in comparison to isolated architectures, the authentication of the integral parts of an MCC architecture has drawn the attention of academic and commercial circles [6].

A few studies [7 - 11] analyzed and/or proposed authentication solutions for MCC environments, which indicates the existence of many widely used authentication methods and protocols globally recognized by researchers and even standardized by some regulatory bodies. Among such methods, some biometric techniques have proved interesting alternatives, not only because they depend exclusively on intrinsic human aspects to be authenticated, but also because they enable the continuity of authentication (the user can remain authenticated throughout the session [12] in a transparent or non-intrusive manner), and authentication at an early stage of a session or transaction (*e.g.*, access of user′s equipment to the MCC infrastructure).

Electrocardiography-based biometrics is one such option. Its characteristics are unique, hardly falsified, can be measured, and are exhibited with no individual′s voluntary intervention, or intervention by an individual from whom they are extracted [13 - 15]. Therefore, the method can be used in activities of authentication of individuals by automated information systems.

Although electrocardiography is a good option for authentication, the misinterpretation of data from electrocardiograms (ECGs) can lead to distortions. Machine learning (ML) [16] has shown a flexible and robust alternative for minimizing such a problem since it provides good solutions to complex classification issues and effectiveness and efficiency for authentication.

ML techniques include ensembles (*e.g.*, AdaBoost, Robust Boost, Random Forest), which represent a strategy according to which multiple simple learners are trained and then used in combination [17]. They can provide a better performance, in terms of precision, sensitivity, and accuracy, in comparison to that of the best simple classifier from the set used individually, and in many cases, to that of different and more complex classifiers trained under other strategies [18]. Consequently, they have been used in several tasks involving signal and data classification, such as voice recognition [19], adaptive face recognition [20], and brain degenerative diseases diagnoses [21].

This chapter introduces a non-intrusive and continuous authentication protocol for MCC environments, and reports on its evaluation regarding effectiveness and efficiency, as well as a comparative analysis with other schemes from the literature. Machine learning techniques that provide levels of appropriate accuracy, precision and sensitivity are addressed from characteristics extracted from temporal analysis and amplitude of the ECG signal. Our protocol is inserted in a Cyber-physical System (CPS) since it integrates physical and software components towards monitoring vital signs and using them as a method of authentication of individuals by systems.

On the other hand, we use Adaptative Boost (Adaboost) and Random Undersampling Boost (RUSBoost), two ensemble-type ML techniques that rely on boosting algorithms for classification after supervised training stages, which can provide comparatively high performance even from relatively few training examples than others ML techniques.

The protocol is based on fiducial points, which are specific and relevant points of the cardiac signal, here used for the obtaining of temporal and amplitude-based inter-point distances to be adopted as part of the user identification process. The detection of such fiducial points is of great importance for the success of the ECG- based authentication process [22]. Moreover, the normalization of temporal inter-point distances of ECG signals should be investigated towards improvements in the classification process based on ML techniques.

Below are the main contributions of this chapter:

• Proposal of an authentication protocol based on analyses of ECG signals and ML techniques;

• Use of RUSBoost for the classification of electrocardiographic signals for user authentication, with better results than Adaboost.

The chapter is organized as follows: Section 2 briefly describes and compares some articles on the themes explored in this research; Section 3 presents the authentication protocol with its several phases, methods and algorithms used; Section 4 is devoted to the evaluation of the protocol focusing on aspects related to electrocardiography and machine learning techniques; finally, Section 5 provides the conclusions and suggests some future work.

RELATED WORK

Some previous studies evaluate the use of electrocardiography (ECG) signals for authentication, with potential applications in MCC environments. These studies include different authentication schemes, models, and protocols, but they can be grouped into two main categories. The first is that of studies that start the ECG analysis by extracting the so-called fiducial points, related to ECG peaks and valleys, by using different types of automatic or semi-automatic algorithms. In these studies, the authors then compute temporal features based on the fiducial points, leading to the inputs based on which the authentication takes place. The other category is that of studies that either use other types of feature extraction, without relying on the detection of fiducial points, or which do not use an explicit feature extraction stage. In the latter case, the authors leave to the classifier the task of analyzing the full time-domain ECG representation, before taking the final decision regarding the user's authenticity.

In our proposed authentication method, we chose the fiducial points-based approach, since we can then use explicit normalization algorithms to compensate for changes in ECG signals due to normal rate variability [22]. Amongst the mentioned studies, however, we emphasize four recent publications. The first is by D. Rezgui and Z. Lachiri [14], who proposed the use of 10 morphological features related to ECG, besides 21 fiducial point-based features. They reach a final authentication accuracy of 99.38%. A second work, by Arteaga-Falconi *et al.* [13], uses 8 features based on fiducial points, from ECG signals, leading to an accuracy of 81.82%, by using a Nearest-Neighbor Search (NNS) classifier. The authors claim that their paper is the first-ever published on mobile authentication based on ECG signals. The third work we emphasize is that by Camara *et al.* [15], in which the authors propose machine learning and data mining models for ECG-based authentication. They use a non-fiducial approach to feature extraction, in which they compute the Walsh-Hadamard transform of the input signals and discard similar values. They then obtain an accuracy of 94.79%, by applying the k-Nearest Neighbors (kNN) classifier to the obtained features. Finally, Arteaga-Falconi *et al.*, [23] advance their previous work [13] by replacing the NNS with a Support Vector Machine (SVM). They claim to reach an accuracy of 100%, but they use fingerprint-based authentication in addition to the ECG signals, thus requiring a process that is no longer non-intrusive.

Besides the related works that were addressed and are based on ECG signals for authentication, this section details some articles related to authentication schemes, protocols, or models used for authentication in MCC environments.

Efficient Privacy-Aware Authentication Scheme for Mobile Cloud Computing Services

A privacy-aware authentication (PAA) scheme is proposed to solve the MCC environments' identification problem [24].

An interesting feature of PAA systems is that the participants' identities can be protected, making it possible to guarantee the privacy of this data, which, for certain situations, proves to be an important aspect in the context of MCC.

A previously proposed scheme [25] is analyzed, and questions are indicated that demonstrate that this scheme, in addition to being insecure against the attack of "impersonation before a service provider," does not make it possible to guarantee users' anonymity.

The authors then propose a new scheme that solves the problems observed in the previous model, based on the use of smart cards, identity-based signatures, and bilinear pairing, using a password and fingerprint as an option to protect the parameters stored on the smart card.

For the new scheme, a network model is proposed, in which the entities "User," "Cloud Service Provider (CSP)," and "Smart Card Generator (SCG)" are present and in which users and CSPs will perform mutual authentication. The phasing of the proposed scheme is based on three steps:

• System configuration phase - the SCG is configured by choosing parameters that will be used in the following phases;

• Registration phase - users and CSPs register with the SCG and obtain their private keys that will be used in the next phase;

• Authentication phase - users and CSP authenticate each other and generate a session key that will be used to ensure the security of their message exchanges.

After presenting the new scheme, the authors present the security model and analyze the compliance with the following security requirements: mutual authentication, user anonymity, non-traceability, key establishment, known session key security, perfect forward secrecy, no check table, no clock synchronization. Also, they show that the scheme is resistant to attacks: inside attack, stolen card attack, repeat attack, impersonation, CSP spoofing, stolen check table attack, a man in the middle.

Finally, a performance analysis is carried out focusing on computing and communication costs.

The scheme proposed [24], despite considering several important aspects to avoid the indicated attacks, including fingerprint-based biometrics, does not guarantee that the user remains continuously authenticated before the CSP. For example, if a user uses a computer to perform his initial authentication and leaves this equipment for a while, an intruder will have the ability to gain access to the services that would be directed to the authenticated user.

In this context, the initial authentication using a fingerprint was insufficient to maintain security in a continuous manner, which is one of the critical characteristics of the protocol proposed in this book chapter.

An Enhanced Privacy-Aware Authentication Scheme for Distributed Mobile Cloud Computing Services

An enhanced privacy-aware Single Sign-On (SSO) scheme is proposed to carry out the identification processes in distributed MCC services [26].

This scheme allows mutual authentication without the aid of an online registration centre; it is resistant to several known attacks ("wrong password attack", "impersonation attack") it makes possible the users' anonymity and perfect forward secrecy, besides presenting advantages in performance terms (computational and communication cost) when compared to other similar schemes.

The scheme is based on the use of bilinear pairing, considers four entities (the user, his mobile device (MD), the registration centre (RC), which represents a trusted third party (TTP), and the service provider (SP)) and is described in five stages:

• Initialization phase - RC uses bilinear pairing to create a private key and its linked parameters for the exchange of messages that will occur later with users;

• User registration phase - the user registers before RC by sending and receiving parameters;

• Service provider registration phase - the service provider registers before RC in a similar way to the previous phase;

• Authentication phase - mutual authentication of the user and the service provider takes place using the parameters obtained and calculated from the previous three phases and, in the end, a session key is generated that will guarantee security for the exchanges of messages that will occur between the user and the SP;

• Password change phase - occurs when the user wants to change his password and takes place on the user's equipment (the other entities are not involved).

It is interesting to note that, to protect secret parameters used by users during the described phases, only passwords created by the users are used (biometrics or data stored on a smart card are not used).

After the description, security and performance analyzes are carried out. A security model is defined from which a formal demonstration of the security existing in the scheme's use is carried out. Besides, it is stated that the proposition is resistant to attacks "from inside", "stolen checker", "repetition", "user impersonation", "man in the middle", "wrong login/change password", is based on two-factor security, provides mutual authentication, anonymity, non-traceability, and perfect forward secrecy.

In the end, performance comparisons are made with other schemes proposed in the existing literature.

The observation made to the previous work is also relevant for this work, as it does not present ways to enable continuous authentication as the proposal of this book chapter. The fact that bimodal authentication is used is positive; however, the non-use of biometric characteristics allows an attacker, in possession of a smart card and password, stolen from a user, to access the services to which he should not have access.

CC Authentication Service Based on Keystroke Standards

A new authentication system is proposed based on the keystroke dynamics on conventional keyboards and touchscreen keyboards, an example of the application of behavioural biometrics to increase the strength of the authentication of users of computational cloud services [27]. The system architecture considers two phases:

• User registration phase - in which data acquisition is performed using the keyboard (conventional or touchscreen), the extraction of keystroke characteristics, a clustering to facilitate the future search in the database authentication, and storage on this database;

• User login phase - where conventional credentials (username and password) are used to verify the user. If the verification is positive, the biometric characteristics are extracted for comparison with the content stored on the authentication database.

In the rest of the work, a detailed analysis is made of obtaining and analyzing the biometric characteristics that will be used in the authentication process.

A comment that can be made regarding the proposed architecture is that it does not use "something that the user has" (a smart card or a token, for example), one of the categories whose use should focus on strong authentication methods. The chosen behavioural biometry technique, despite being able to achieve continuous user authentication, presents issues when applied to authentication to content providers that do not require many user interactions (*e.g.,* video and music providers) [28].

Efficient Authentication System Based on Several Factors For MCC

A new authentication system is proposed based on several factors (user and password, voice recognition, face recognition, international mobile equipment identity (IMEI), an international mobile subscriber identity (IMSI)) to provide security efficiently in mobile cloud computing environments [29].

One of the interesting aspects of the protocol is that the analyses of each of the factors used for authentication are carried out on different virtual machines provided by the computing cloud environment, making it possible to parallelize the process and improve its efficiency.

Before describing the system itself, the paper indicates some information security considerations that need to be observed for an MCC. It suggests using hybrid computational clouds (partly public, partly private) to provide adequate security to the various types of existing data. It also indicates safety aspects that must be observed in mobile equipment used in the MCC environment.

The system architecture has the following characteristics:

• The five authentication factors (user/password, voice, face, IMEI, and IMSI) captured by the user's mobile device are subjected to a hash function inside the device;

• The communication between the mobile equipment and the cloud environment is protected by conventional security protocols used in wireless networks (Wi-Fi Protected Access 2 (WPA2), *etc.*) and transactions *via* the Internet (Secure Socket Layer (SSL) / Transport Layer Security (TLS), *etc.*);

• The data for each of the authentication factors considered are stored in separate areas of the authentication database;

• Each factor is analyzed in a specific virtual machine to increase efficiency.

The operation of the system takes place in two phases, in which the entities "user equipment," "management server," "storage area," and "processing area" participate:

• Registration - the five authentication factors are extracted (the user's equipment or others that enable the appropriate extraction of the necessary characteristics can be used) and stored in the storage area (the data to be inserted must be compared to those already stored so that possible redundancies can be blocked);

• Authentication - the five factors are captured from the user's equipment (using the sensors and other components of the device itself) and are sent to the five virtual machines responsible for the comparison processes to be carried out between captured data and stored data; if all processes indicate success in their comparisons, the authentication process will be completed successfully, otherwise, if there is any wrong comparison, authentication will fail.

After describing the new system, the authors present abbreviated analyzes of security and performance using comparisons with other similar works.

The proposed system has some parts that can be considered unnecessary. IMEI and IMSI use as authentication factors can be seen as something redundant (and for this reason, which violates aspects of efficiency) since both represent a "one has" authentication factor. Besides, IMEI prevents the user from using other equipment to access the services provided by the CSP. If the option was to use only the IMEI (as the protocol proposed in this book chapter), the user could use any equipment, as the IMEI is on the chip that can be passed from one device to another.

Regarding the types of biometric authentication used (voice and face recognition), these have disadvantages (as indicated in the next section) concerning electrocardiography, which is the option adopted in this book chapter.

Comparison Between the Works Presented and this Work

Table **1** presents a comparison between the different schemes, protocols, and models presented and the protocol proposed in this work.

Table 1. Comparison between the general works analyzed.

Characteristics	[24]	[26]	[27]	[29]	Proposal of this Work
Cloud type	MCC	MCC	CC	MCC	MCC
Mutual authentication	Yes	Yes	No	No	Yes
Continuous authentication	No	No	Yes	Yes	Yes
Smart card / identity card	Yes	No	No	Yes	Yes
Requires TTP	No	Yes	Yes	No	No
Authentication factors	Password, fingerprint	Password	Password, typing analysis	Password, speech recognition, facial recognition, IMSI, IMEI	Password, ECG, IMSI

PROPOSED PROTOCOL

Initial Considerations

This section introduces a protocol for a non-intrusive and continuous authentication of users of MCC environments which uses the following three factors:

• "something the person knows" - a password;

• "something the person has" - a card with the Subscriber Identity Module (SIM) containing an IMSI; and

• "something intrinsic to the person" - their cardiac cycles represented by an electrocardiogram.

The use of a password is the simplest way to represent the first category of factors. Since this technique will be combined with other mechanisms, the effects of the vulnerabilities cited in the theoretical basis tend to be minimized. The rules for the creation of the password are not subject to in-depth analysis, and a standard with a minimum size of eight alphanumeric characters (upper- and lower-case letters, numbers, and symbols obtained from a common keyboard) is generated from the UE interface is adopted.

Regarding the use of IMSI, a different alternative would be the application of IMEI. However, it would relate the authentication process to some specific equipment, thus decreasing the flexibility of the system by restricting the user's authentication to that equipment and causing security problems of loss or theft of the equipment. IMSI promotes user authentication from any equipment of appropriate characteristics and presence of IMSI.

The use of cardiac cycles data (present in the ECG) as biometric features of authentication can be considered a non-intrusive and transparent technique to the user (the placement of a cardiac chest sensor, for example, can be similar to the use of a simple cardiac strap monitor commonly used by athletes, and can provide the necessary data for the creation of a representative ECG for the authentication process). It offers security advantages over other biometric techniques, such as voice recognition, subject to an attack based on the reproduction of a recording of the user's voice, facial recognition, subject to an attack based on the presentation of a captured image of the user, and fingerprint recognition, which cannot be considered transparent to the user.

Still, regarding electrocardiography, the biometric features will be classified by machine learning techniques (ML).

It is important to note that, in addition to the factors aimed at user authentication before the CSP, this provider is also authenticated against the user using a digital certificate found at the CSP itself. Therefore, our protocol can be considered mutual authentication between user and provider. In the models presented below, this aspect will be represented, in a simplified way, by an SSL / TLS connection created based on the CSP digital certificate and that protects the existing data flows between the provider and the user's mobile equipment.

The Network Model

Fig. (**2**) shows the network model in which our authentication protocol should work.

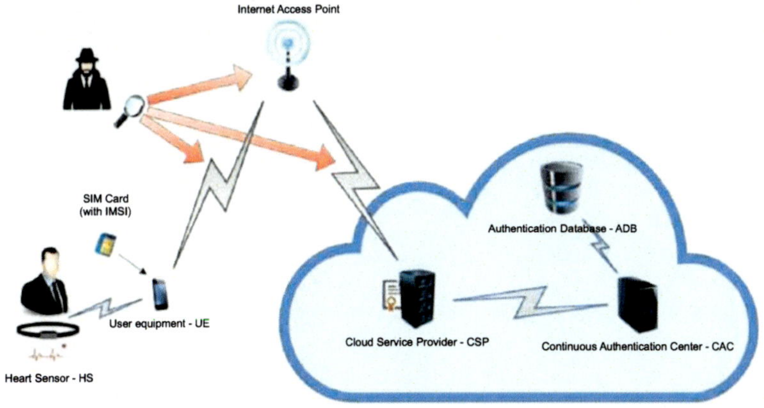

Fig. (2). Network model considered.

The main entities are:

• Cardiac (heart) sensor (HS), which captures the user's cardiac signals for the creation of an ECG representative of the individual;

• User equipment (UE), through which the user authenticates and receives the services made available by the service provider;

• Cloud Computing Service Provider (CSP), which centralizes requests and provision of cloud computing services. It must verify the authenticity of the plaintiffs (users) and authenticate itself (as reported elsewhere, the CSP for this model has a digital certificate linked to asymmetric cryptographic keys that enables its authentication with users);

• Continuous Authentication Center (CAC), which is a set of entities (real or virtual machines) of the computational cloud allocated for the various tasks related to the authentication processes; and

• Authentication Database (ADB), which stores data to be used in authentication processes.

The protocol aims at an end-to-end authentication and is designed to work at the application layer; several communication technologies can be used in the lower layers. For instance, the HS can communicate with the UE through a Bluetooth connection, the UE can communicate with the CSP through an Internet connection *via* WLAN or cellular networks (*e.g.,* 3G, 4G, 5G), and the internal entities of the cloud can communicate using the technologies available in the cloud (*e.g.,* Ethernet connections that use different cables, optical fibres or even establish wireless communications).

The communication channels considered insecure and, therefore, subject to the action of possible attackers or intruders, are located between the UE and the CSP, as shown in Fig. (**2**), where a potential attacker is monitoring the indicated channels. The other environments (region close to the user where HS and UE are present, and internal cloud environment formed by CSP, CAC, and ADB) are considered free from threats.

The Authentication Model

The proposed authentication protocol is divided into the following three phases:

• Registration, in which the user introduces himself to the system and has some of his data collected (*e.g.,* password, IMSI, and raw electrocardiographic signals) and stored for the following phases.

• Authentication (initial or continuous), in which the user presents fresh data that, after being compared with those already stored, generate the acceptance or rejection of the user's access.

• Update (in a controlled environment or during an authenticated session), in which new data replace those stored in the registration phase.

Algorithm **1** provides an overview of the operation of the authentication protocol, detailed in the following items.

Algorithm 1. General operation of the proposed authentication protocol.

```
START
    Select Phase
        Phase = Registration
            User provides Set = {Password, IMSI and Raw ECG Data}
                                                        to CSP
            CSP forwards Set to CAC
            CAC extracts ECG features and trains the classifier
            CAC stores in ADB the data necessary for user authentication
                    (IMSI, password hash and trained classifier parameters)
        Phase = Initial Authentication
            User provides Set = {Password, IMSI and Raw ECG Data} to CSP
            CSP forwards Set to CAC
            CAC extracts ECG features and authenticates the user using
password,
                                        IMSI and trained classifier
        Phase = Continuous Authentication
            User provides raw ECG data to CSP
            CSP forwards raw ECG data to CAC
            CAC extracts ECG features and authenticates the user using the
                                              trained classifier
        Phase = Update in a controlled environment
            User provides Set' = {new Password, IMSI and Raw ECG
                                                        data} to CSP
            CSP forwards Set' to CAC
            CAC extracts ECG features and trains the classifier
            CAC updates, in the ADB, the data necessary for the user
                          authentication (new password hash and
                                  trained classifier parameters)
        Phase = Update during an authenticated session
            User provides Set'' = {new Password and Raw ECG Data}
                                                        to CSP
            CSP forwards Set'' to CAC
            CAC extracts ECG features and trains the classifier
            CAC updates, in the ADB, the data necessary for the user
                          authentication (new password hash and
                                  trained classifier parameters)
    End of Selection
END
```

Registration

In this phase, performed before the protocol starts authentication, relevant user´s data (ECG, IMSI, and Password) are captured and sent to the cloud to be stored in the ADB for future authentication processes. The phase must be triggered in a controlled physical environment where the CSP is secure regarding the user's identity.

Continuous capture of raw ECG data is foreseen until the minimum necessary number of cycles recognized for classifier training has been obtained and the recording phase has been completed.

The sequence diagram in Fig. (**3**) represents the Registration phase, which is divided into the following steps:

• The UE receives a password (*Pwd*) registered directly by the user, the IMSI obtained from the SIM Card, and the raw ECG data extracted from the user *via* HS;

• Using the CSP digital certificate, the UE creates an SSL connection between itself and the CSP through which all data (IMSI, password hash - H (Pwd) and raw ECG data) are sent;

• The CSP receives the data through the SSL connection and forwards it to the CAC, which verifies the existence of the IMSI is included in the ADB;

• If the IMSI is not found, the CAC processes the raw ECG data by recognizing their cycles, detecting the fiducial points, and extracting the ECG features to be used in the authentication process;

• ECG features are then used for training the classifier, which then provides its training parameters to be stored in the ADB and used in the authentication processes;

• After all such processes have succeeded, CAC registers all data (IMSI, H (Pwd), and the classifier parameters) in the ADB.

It must be emphasized that any event that escapes the processes represented in the phase diagrams (*e.g.,* the previous existence of an IMSI being registered, or a failure in the classifier training process) will automatically interrupt the phase being triggered and establish an adequate communication for the parties involved and the return to the context before the execution of the phase.

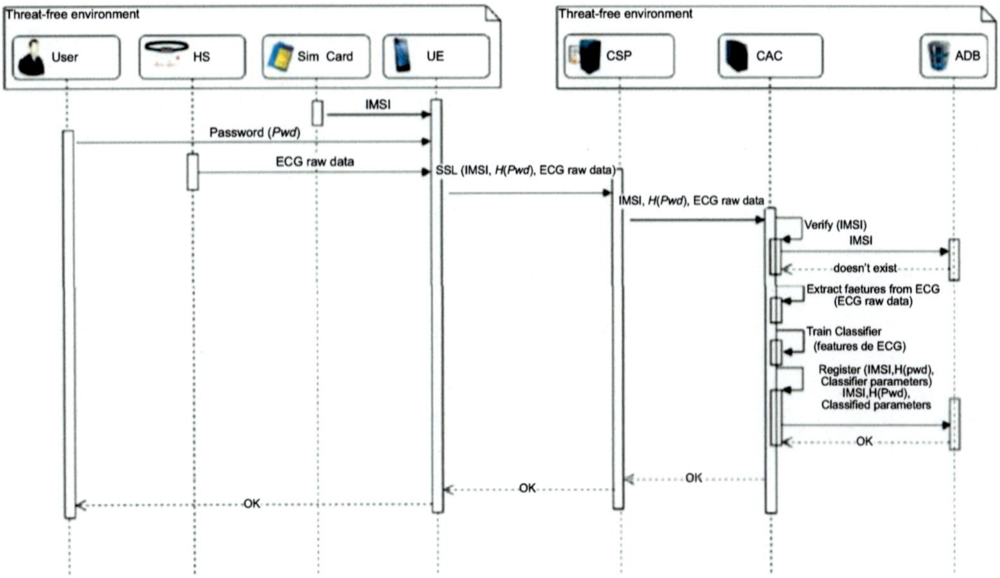

Fig. (3). Registration phase.

Authentication

A phase that occurs whenever a user wishes to authenticate with the CSP for requesting a service. It is divided into two subphases:

• Initial authentication - the user submits his credentials to the CSP to be authenticated at the beginning of a secure communication session between them; and

• Continuous authentication - after initial authentication, the user who wishes to remain authenticated by the CSP continuously sends (iteratively) his raw ECG data to the CAC.

Initial Authentication

The sequence diagram in Fig. (**4**) represents the initial authentication subphase, which is divided into the following steps:

• The UE receives the password typed directly by the user, the IMSI obtained from the SIM Card, and raw ECG data extracted from the user through cardiac sensors (HS);

• Using the CSP digital certificate, the UE creates an SSL connection between it and the CSP through which the IMSI, H (Pwd), and raw ECG data are sent;

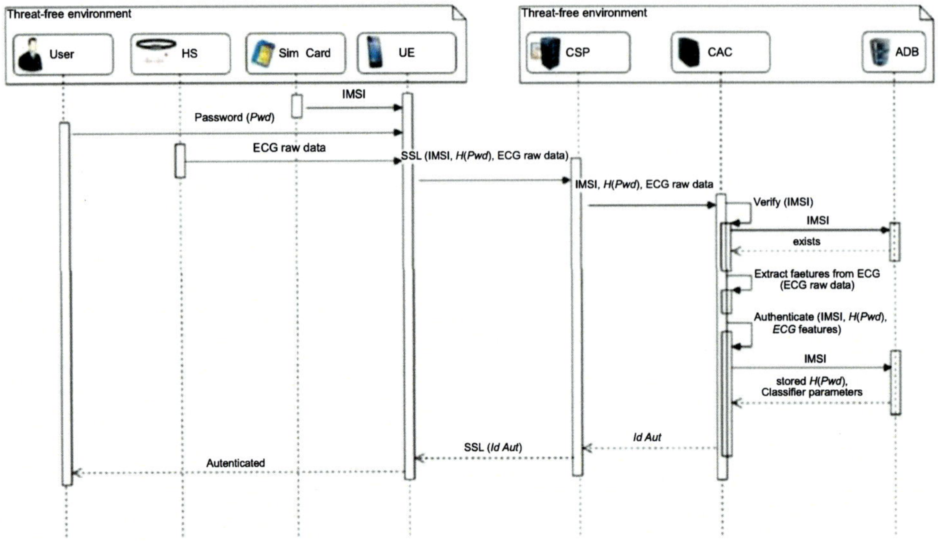

Fig. (4). Initial authentication subphase.

- The CSP forwards the data received to the CAC;
- The CAC verifies the existence of the IMSI in the ADB;
- If the IMSI is found, the CAC processes the raw ECG data by extracting the ECG features to be used in the authentication process;
- The CAC then authenticates the user by comparing the H (Pwd) received with the H (Pwd) stored in the ADB and classifying the extracted ECG features using the classifier trained with the parameters stored in the ADB;
- If the password hash comparison and classification confirm the authenticity of the user, the CAC creates an authentication identifier (IdAut) for a secure communication session between the CSP and the user;
- The CAC sends the IdAut to the CSP, which forwards it to the UE *via* SSL, signalling the initial authentication was successful and that the user can now access the services to be provided by the CSP.

It should be noted that, for both initial and continuous authentication, each classification performed by the ML algorithm using ECG features is performed on data equivalent to one cardiac cycle verified on the electrocardiogram. Therefore, the raw ECG data extracted from the user must be sufficient for this complete cycle to be recognized.

Continuous Authentication

The continuous authentication sub-phase is performed iteratively, after the initial authentication, as long as the user wishes to remain authenticated before the CSP. At this point, a secure communication session has been established between the CSP and the user identified by IdAut.

The sequence diagram in Fig. (**5**) represents an iteration of the continuous authentication subphase in which the following steps are taken:

• The UE receives the raw ECG data extracted from the user through cardiac sensors;

• IdAut and raw ECG data are sent through the SSL connection established between the UE and the CSP;

• The CSP forwards the data received to the CAC;

• The CAC processes the raw ECG data by extracting the ECG features to be used in the authentication process;

• The CAC authenticates the user by classifying the newly obtained ECG features with the trained classifier;

• The CAC confirms the success of the continuous authentication iteration and returns the IdAut to the CSP, which forwards it to the user, signalling he can access the services.

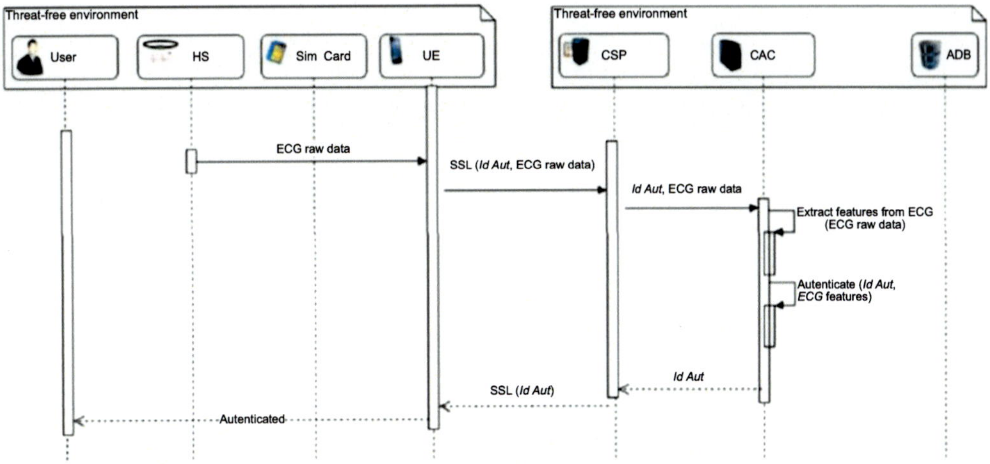

Fig. (5). An iteration of the continuous authentication subphase.

It is important to note that continuous authentication is performed using each cardiac cycle. In this context, two situations deserve special attention: the protocol does not recognize any cycle (and, consequently, cannot use them for authentication), and the protocol refutes the authentication of some cycle. Since the proposed model is multifactorial, it has a relevant level of security, which is independent of biometric authentication, since there are two other factors. Therefore, the authenticated session is not interrupted immediately after the occurrence of one of the situations. The protocol considers the following alternatives for such cases:

• If a cycle is not recognized, new attempts are made successively after the failure and, if the problem remains longer than a predefined tolerance, the session is interrupted, and its restart is requested (the process proceeds normally if the cycles are recognized before the time of tolerance).

• If any cycle is disproved in authentication, similarly to the previous situation, new attempts are made towards reversing the problem (if it is reversed, the process proceeds normally). If a maximum tolerance time is reached, the session is interrupted and authentication is locked - it is unlocked only after an update in a controlled environment (explained in what follows).

Update

This phase is performed when a change must be made to one or more data linked to the user stored in the ADB. It is motivated by the forgetting of a password, a change in the cardiac pattern (caused by surgery, for example), and a need (or desire) to change a password or retrain the classifier. Since the IMSI is the basis for user identification, such data cannot be modified in the update - the IMSI is changed if a new phase of user registration has been triggered.

The update is performed in two ways:

• In a controlled environment, when the user is no longer able to authenticate with the CSP (forgetting a password, changing the cardiac authentication pattern, *etc.*) and, as in the registration phase, must be triggered in a controlled physical environment, where the CSP is sure about the user's identity; and

• During an authenticated session, when the user wishes to change his password and/or retrain the classifier.

Update in a Controlled Environment

The sequence diagram in Fig. (**6**) represents the update in a controlled environment, where the following steps are taken:

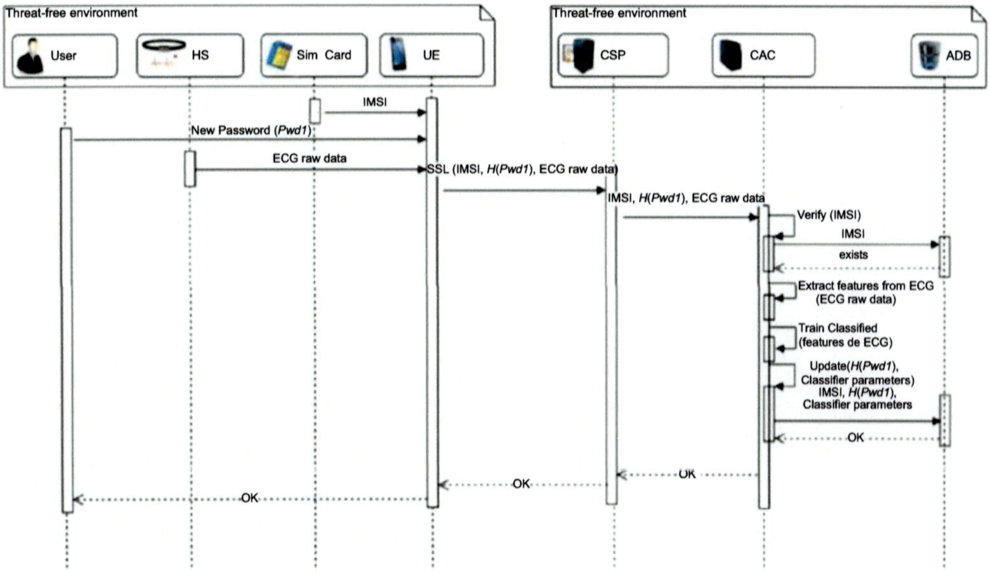

Fig. (6). Update phase in a controlled environment.

• The UE receives the data to be changed (the new password - Pwd1 - and the raw ECG data) and the current IMSI;

• The CSP forwards the data received to the CAC;

• The CAC verifies the existence of the IMSI presented in the ADB;

• If the IMSI is found, the CAC processes the raw ECG data by extracting the ECG features to be used in the authentication process (as in the registration, more data must be provided in case of insufficient raw ECG data for the training of the classifier);

• ECG features are then used for the training of the classifier, which then provides its training parameters to be stored in the ADB and further used in the authentication processes;

• The CAC updates the data recorded in the ADB by modifying H (Pwd1) and the classifier parameters;

• The CAC informs both CSP and user on the successful change.

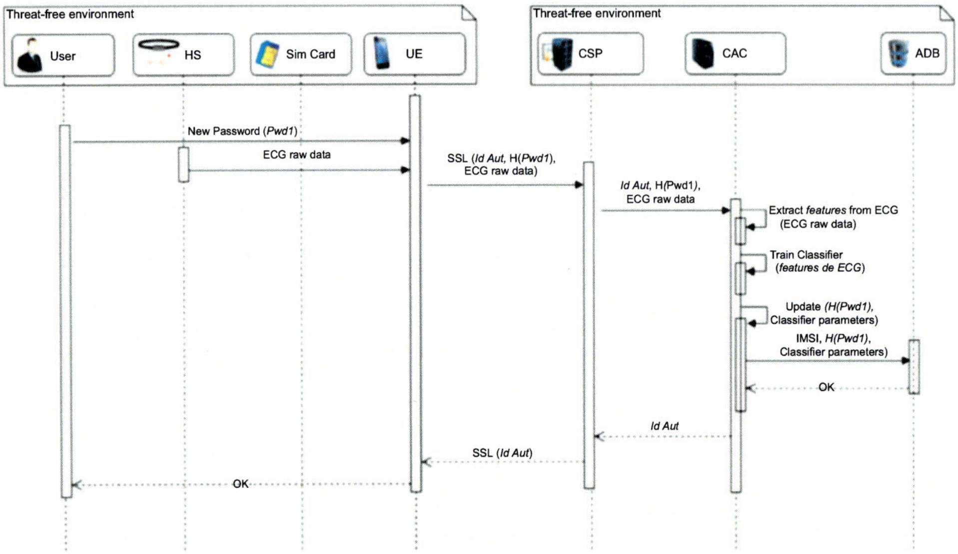

Fig. (7). Update phase during an authenticated session.

Update During an Authenticated Session

As reported before, the update is performed when the user is authenticated before the CSP. The sequence diagram in Fig. (**7**) represents the update during an authenticated session in which the following steps are taken:

• The UE receives the data to be changed (the new password - Pwd1 - and the raw ECG data);

• IdAut, H (Pwd1) and raw ECG data are sent through the SSL connection established between the UE and the CSP;

• The CSP forwards the data received to the CAC;

• The CAC processes the raw ECG data by extracting the ECG features to be used in the authentication process (more data must be provided, like previous phases);

• ECG features are then used for the training of the classifier, which then provides its training parameters to be stored in the ADB;

• The CAC updates the data recorded in the ADB by modifying H (Pwd1) and the classifier parameters;

• The CAC informs both CSP and user on the successful change and proceeds with the authenticated session.

Specific Aspects of the Electrocardiography-Based Process

Below are some aspects related to electrocardiography:

• The proposal focuses on the authentication of individuals with no cardiac abnormalities and whose cardiac cycles follow a certain pattern (indicated below). This premise is mainly used for imposing conditions for the detection of fiducial points used in the extraction of features. If it is not adopted, the fiducial point detection algorithm used must follow another logic of operation, which is outside the scope of this research;

• The cardiac cycle adopted is a curve representing part of an ECG between a fiducial point LP and the subsequent fiducial point TP, *i.e.,* a waveform containing fiducial points LP, P, Q, R, S, T, and TP, which are the basis for the extraction process of ECG features (Fig. **8**). The cycle must follow a pattern according to which, from a fiducial point, the path to the next point must exhibit only one behaviour, *i.e.,* be ascending or descending (the path may contain horizontal segments);

• Although the fiducial point detection algorithm developed is based on the indicated pattern, it has some tolerance ranges that enable the recognition of a cycle even if shows small (configurable) variations in the desired behaviour.

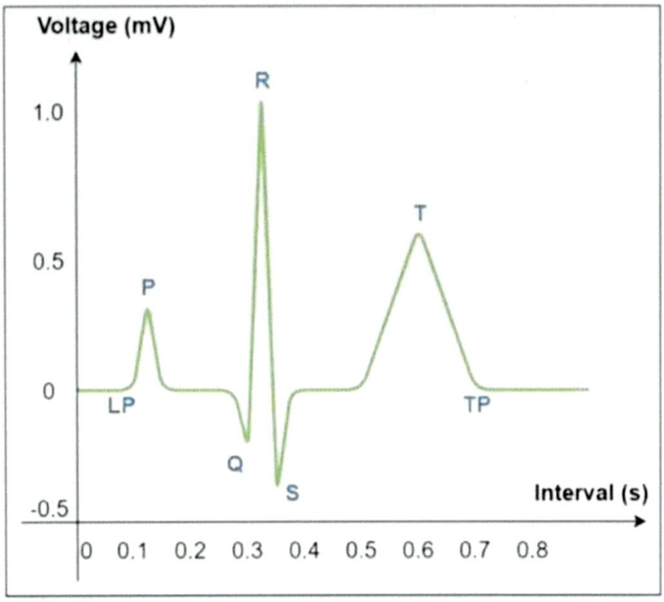

Fig. (8). Typical cardiac cycle.

The treatment of data derived from ECG consists of the following three main methods:

- Extraction of ECG features (including fiducial points detection);
- Training of the classifier; and
- Authentication.

Results Analyses from Electrocardiography-Based Authentication Process

A repository with 108 users developed by [30] was used as an ECG database. During the initial analyses of this ECG database's quality, the researchers concluded that it was quite variable (probably due to cardiac problems of the participants or problems in the capture of electrical signals). It hampered the detection of fiducial points by the extraction of features, thus causing several of such points not to be detected and forcing the cycles to which they belong to be considered unrecognized and discarded from the analyses.

From those 108 users, 37 had 300 cardiac cycles recognized in their ECG (each ECG contained in the repository is at least 5 minutes long) and were chosen to calculate the averages of the metrics presented below. This process was based on the "holdout method" [31] and consisted of the execution of 100 validation sessions formed, each by training the classifiers using 70% of all user's cycles and by the classification (authentication) using the remaining 30%.

Table **2** shows the results of the averages and standards deviations of the metrics obtained at the end of the authentication process:

Table 2. Values of the analysis metrics and the standard deviations.

Classifier	Accuracy ± σ			Precision ± σ			Sensitivity ± σ			F1-Score ± σ		
Ada	0,920	±	0,032	0,962	±	0,038	0,840	±	0,064	0,893	±	0,052
RUS	0.974	±	0.012	0.987	±	0.010	0.961	±	0.022	0.974	±	0.012

According to the proposed model, the analysis metrics presented indicate that the proposed use of ECG for authentication is adequate and achieves excellent results when compared to other methods (*e.g.*, [12 - 14, 23]).

CONCLUSION

User authentication in mobile cloud computing environments represents a challenge. Several protocols have been developed towards overcoming it, and those based on biometric authentication have excelled since they enable the use of data intrinsic to the human being who intends to use the services of a given provider.

This article has addressed a proposal and a partial evaluation of a multi-modal protocol that uses three factors (password, IMSI, biometric signals based on electrocardiograms) to provide mutual authentication to users and CSP.

Signal processing and machine learning techniques were applied to a population of 108 users, of whom 37 were chosen to validate the authentication process because they had 300 cardiac cycles recognized. A protocol that acts on an MCC architecture in an integrated manner and performs operations in a non-intrusive and continuous way, thus improving information security, was obtained.

We have also evaluated the use of the RUSBoost classifier as the main method for processing the ECG extracted features and providing the final result of the whole authentication scheme. The RUSBoost classifier is known for its relative robustness to dataset imbalances, given its use of the boosting strategy combined with random undersampling at each training state. Considering that in authentication, we typically have fewer data collected from any single user than from all the others combined, such robustness is a requirement for proper performance.

Our dataset includes 108 users, so that the complete use of the dataset for training and testing (with different signal samples for each phase) leads to an imbalance of more than 100 times. The other option would be to reduce the imbalance by eliminating training examples, but this can reduce the classifier's generalization power and lead to overfitting. The RUSBoost, on the other hand, allows us to use the whole set of signal samples while avoiding the pitfalls of imbalance.

Our results suggest that, even under such strong imbalance, we can attain performances of over 95%, in terms of accuracy, sensitivity, precision, and F1-measure, by using RUSBoost over the proposed ECG features with cycle normalization. This approach outperformed the ADABoost classifier to the four considered metrics, even though ADABoost also uses the boosting approach, but without random undersampling at the training stages. Under the evaluated conditions, random undersampling improved all evaluated classifier aspects.

These metrics indicate that the proposed protocols and classification strategies provide a reliable solution to the continuous authentication problem so that the user can perform his or her tasks while the system verifies for authenticity in a non-intrusive manner.

CONSENT FOR PUBLICATION

Not applicable

CONFLICT OF INTEREST

The author declares no conflict of interest, financial or otherwise.

ACKNOWLEDGEMENTS

The authors thank Mr. Pedro Henrique de Brito Souza for authorizing access and use of the ECG database used in this work.

REFERENCES

[1] J. Wan, Z. Liu, K. Zhou, and R. Lu, "Mobile Cloud Computing: Application Scenarios and Service Models", IWCMC - 9th International Wireless Communications and Mobile Computing Conference, 2013.

[2] Q. Jiang, J. Ma, and F. Wei, *On the security of a privacy-aware authentication scheme for distributed mobile cloud computing services* IEEE Systems Journal, 2016, p. 99.

[3] H.T. Dinh, C. Lee, D. Niyato, and P. Wang, *A survey of mobile cloud computing: architecture, applications, and approaches.* vol. 13. Wireless Communication Mobile Computing, 2013.

[4] H. Suo, Z. Liu, J. Wan, and K. Zhou, "Security and privacy in mobile Cloud Computing", IWCMC - 9th International Wireless Communications and Mobile Computing Conference, 2013. [http://dx.doi.org/10.1109/IWCMC.2013.6583635]

[5] M.D. Ryan, "Cloud computing security: The scientific challenge, and a survey of solutions", *J. Syst. Softw.,* vol. 86, no. 9, pp. 2263-2268, 2013. [http://dx.doi.org/10.1016/j.jss.2012.12.025]

[6] M. Alizadeh, S. Abolfazli, M. Zamani, S. Baharun, and K. Sakurai, "Authentication in mobile cloud computing: A survey", *J. Netw. Comput. Appl.,* vol. 61, no. C, pp. 59-80, 2016. [http://dx.doi.org/10.1016/j.jnca.2015.10.005]

[7] D. He, N. Kumar, M.K. Khan, L. Wang, and J. Shen, "Efficient Privacy-Aware Authentication Scheme for Mobile Cloud Computing Services", *IEEE Syst. J.,* vol. 12, no. 2, pp. 1621-1631, 2018. [http://dx.doi.org/10.1109/JSYST.2016.2633809]

[8] J. Mohsin, "Two Factor *vs.* Multi-Factor, an Authentication Battle in Mobile Cloud Computing Environments", International Conference on Future Networks and Distributed Systems Proceedings, No, vol. 39, 2017. [http://dx.doi.org/10.1145/3102304.3102343]

[9] B. Jannati, "An Improved Authentication Protocol for Distributed Mobile Cloud Computing Services", *International Journal of Critical Infrastructure Protection.,* vol. 19, 2017. [http://dx.doi.org/10.1016/j.ijcip.2017.10.003]

[10] S. Audithan, V. Vijayasaro, P. Vijayakumar, and V. Vijayakumar, "An Efficient Authentication Scheme for Mobile Cloud Computing Services", *J. Inf. Sci. Eng.,* vol. 33, no. 3, 2017.

[11] M. Al-Rubaie, and J.M. Chang, "Reconstruction Attacks Against Mobile-Based Continuous Authentication Systems in the Cloud", *IEEE Trans. Inf. Forensics Security,* vol. 11, no. 12, pp. 2648-2663, 2016. [http://dx.doi.org/10.1109/TIFS.2016.2594132]

[12] A. Mosenia, S. Sur-Kolay, A. Raghunathan, and N.K. Jha, "CABA: Continuous Authentication Based on BioAura", *IEEE Trans. Comput.*, vol. 66, no. 5, pp. 759-772, 2017. [http://dx.doi.org/10.1109/TC.2016.2622262]

[13] J.S. Arteaga-Falconi, H. Al Osman, and A. El Saddik, "ECG Authentication for Mobile Devices", *IEEE Trans. Instrum. Meas.*, vol. 65, no. 3, pp. 591-600, 2016. [http://dx.doi.org/10.1109/TIM.2015.2503863]

[14] D. Rezgui, and Z. Lachiri, "ECG Biometric Recognition Using SVM-Based Approach", *Institute of Electrical Engineers of Japan - Transactions on Electrical and Electronic Engineering,* 2016. [http://dx.doi.org/10.1002/tee.22241]

[15] C. Camara, P. Peris-Lopez, L. Gonzalez-Manzano, and J. Tapiador, "Real-time electrocardiogram streams for continuous authentication", *Appl. Soft Comput.*, vol. 68, pp. 784-794, 2018. [http://dx.doi.org/10.1016/j.asoc.2017.07.032]

[16] O. Simeone, "A Brief Introduction to Machine Learning for Engineers", *Computer Science, Mathematics, Foundations, and Trends in Signal Processing.,* 2017.

[17] Z. Zhou, *Ensemble Methods - Foundations and Algorithms.* 1st ed. Chapman and Hall - CRC, 2012. [http://dx.doi.org/10.1201/b12207]

[18] R. Barandela, R.M. Valdovinos, and J.S. Sánchez, "New Applications of Ensembles of Classifiers", *Pattern Anal. Appl.,* vol. 6, no. 3, pp. 245-256, 2003. [http://dx.doi.org/10.1007/s10044-003-0192-z]

[19] Y. Zhao, J. Xue, and X. Chen, Ensemble Learning Approaches in Speech Recognition.*Speech and Audio Processing for Coding.* Enhancement and Recognition, 2014, pp. 113-152.

[20] C. Pagano, E. Granger, R. Sabourin, G.L. Marcialis, and F. Roli, "Adaptive ensembles for face recognition in changing video surveillance environments", *Inf. Sci.,* vol. 286, pp. 75-101, 2014. [http://dx.doi.org/10.1016/j.ins.2014.07.005]

[21] P. Dai, F. Gwadry-Sridhar, M. Bauer, and M. Borrie, "Bagging Ensembles for the Diagnosis and Prognostication of Alzheimer's Disease", *Thirtieth AAAI Conference on Artificial Intelligence (AAAI-16),* 2016 Phoenix, Arizona, USA [http://dx.doi.org/10.1609/aaai.v30i1.9915]

[22] A. Fratini, M. Sansone, P. Bifulco, and M. Cesarelli, "Individual identification *via* electrocardiogram analysis", Biomed. Eng. Online, vol. 14, no. 1, p. 78, 2015. [http://dx.doi.org/10.1186/s12938-015-0072-y] [PMID: 26272456]

[23] J.S. Arteaga-Falconi, H.A. Osman, and A.E. Saddik, *ECG and Fingerprint Bimodal Authentication.* vol. Vol. 40. Sustainable Cities and Society, 2018.

[24] L. Xiong, F. Li, M. He, Z. Liu, and T. Peng, "An Efficient Privacy-Aware Authentication Scheme with Hierarchical Access Control for Mobile Cloud Computing Services", *IEEE Trans. Cloud Comput.,* pp. 1-1, 2020. [http://dx.doi.org/10.1109/TCC.2020.3029878]

[25] J.L. Tsai, and N.W. Lo, "A Privacy-Aware Authentication Scheme for Distributed Mobile Cloud Computing Services", *IEEE Syst. J.,* vol. 9, no. 3, pp. 805-815, 2015. [http://dx.doi.org/10.1109/JSYST.2014.2322973]

[26] L. Xiong, "An Enhanced Privacy-Aware Authentication Scheme for Distributed Mobile Cloud Computing Services", *Trans. Internet Inf. Syst. (Seoul),* vol. 11, no. 12, 2017.

[27] A. Abo-alian, N.L. Badr, and M.F. Tolba, "Keystroke dynamics-based user authentication service for cloud computing", *Concurr. Comput.,* vol. 28, no. 9, pp. 2567-2585, 2016. [http://dx.doi.org/10.1002/cpe.3718]

[28] H. Lee, J.Y. Hwang, D. Kim, S. Lee, S.H. Lee, and J.S. Shin, *Understanding Keystroke Dynamics for Smartphone Users Authentication and Keystroke Dynamics on Smartphones Built-In Motion Sensors.*

Applied Cryptography and Noise Resistant Data Security, 2018. [http://dx.doi.org/10.1155/2018/2567463]

[29] Y.S. Jeong, J.S. Park, and J.H. Park, "An efficient authentication system of smart device using multi factors in mobile cloud service architecture", *Int. J. Commun. Syst.*, vol. 28, no. 4, pp. 659-674, 2015. [http://dx.doi.org/10.1002/dac.2694]

[30] P.H.B. Souza, Método para estimação da frequência cardíaca e variabilidade cardíaca com base em fotopletismografia por vídeo, 2019.

[31] R. Kohavi, "A Study of Cross-Validation and Bootstrap for Accuracy Estimation and Model Selection", IJCAI - International Joint Conference on Artificial Intelligence, 1995.

CHAPTER 6

Recent Trends in Mobile Computing in Health Care, Challenges and Opportunities

S. Kannadhasan[1,*] and **R. Nagarajan**[2]

[1] *Department of Electronics and Communication Engineering, Study World College of Engineering, Tamilnadu, India*

[2] *Department of Electrical and Electronics Engineering, Gnanamani College of Technology, Tamilnadu, India*

Abstract: This paper provides an analysis of IoT protection and privacy problems, as well as current security strategies, as well as a list of open topics for potential study. The most significant inventions are those that vanish. They become indistinguishable from the structure of daily existence when they weave themselves through it. This Internet of Things idea has begun to transform our modern environment, including a common man's daily existence in society, a world in which machines of all shapes and sizes are produced with "smart" capabilities that enable them to connect and interact not only with other devices but also with humans, share data, make autonomous decisions, and perform useful tasks based on predetermined conditions. With its many implementations, the Internet of Things is now a well-known phenomenon across both horizontal and vertical industries.

Keywords: Autonomous, Healthcare, Internet of Things, Smart, Smart IoT.

INTRODUCTION

The environment is rapidly changing from disconnected networks to pervasive Internet-enabled 'things' capable of communicating with one another and producing data that can be analyzed to obtain useful knowledge. The Internet of Things, a massively integrated digital network system, would enhance everyone's existence, increase company growth, boost government performance, and so on. However, from the standpoint of protection and privacy, this modern reality (IoT) created on the Internet poses new problems. Because of the various requirements and networking stacks involved, traditional protection primitives cannot be explicitly extended to IoT technologies. Along with scalability and heterogeneity

* **Corresponding author S. Kannadhasan:** Department of Electronics and Communication Engineering, Study World College of Engineering, Tamilnadu, India; Tel: +919677565511; E-mail: kannadhasan.ece@gmail.com

Sivakumar R., Dimiter Velev, Basim Alhadidi, S. Vidhya, Sheeja V. Francis and B. Prabadevi (Eds.)

problems, resource-constrained systems like RFIDs and wireless sensor nodes make up a large part of IoT infrastructure. As a result, in such a complex setting, a scalable architecture capable of dealing with protection and privacy concerns is needed. To illustrate how the Internet of Things could impact our everyday lives, consider the following scenario: You walk into the store and get a text message from your refrigerator. Sensors in the dairy aisle warn your grocery cart that you've picked up a milk carton. Your exercise wristband vibrates as you head through the store, taking your vitals and sending the findings to your doctor to change your order. You just step out the door after you've done shopping. When you leave the geophone of the store, your credit card is paid. To avoid collisions, the automobile interacts with other vehicles on the road when you head home. Machine to Machine (M2M) correspondence was the foundation of the Internet of Things (IoT) in its early years. M2M connectivity refers to two computers interacting with each other without the need for human intervention. The networking medium isn't defined, and it may be either wireless or wired. The word “machine-to-machine” (M2M) comes from telephony networks. Different endpoints in these networks required to share details with one another, such as the caller's name. This data was transmitted between the endpoints without the need for a person to start the transmission. M2M is still widely used, especially in the industrial industry, and is sometimes considered a subset of IoT [1-5].

Computing devices embedded in everyday items are connected through the Internet, allowing them to transmit and receive data. Nonetheless, modern IoT network technologies such as e-healthcare and transportation services have expanded this definition during the last decade. The Internet of Things arose from the integration of wireless technology, micro electromechanical systems (MEMS) advances, and digital electronics, resulting in small computers that can detect, calculate, and interact wirelessly. The connection or partnership between humans and machines is becoming increasingly important in the Internet of Things age, as machines get smarter and begin to do more human activities, and in this case, humans [6-10].

The next generation of computing will occur outside of the standard desktop setting. Many of the artifacts that accompany us would be linked in any way under the Internet of Things (IoT) model. This latest task, in which knowledge and communication networks are invisibly integrated in the world around us, would be met by RFID and sensor network technology is shown in Fig. (**1**). As a consequence, massive quantities of data are produced which must be collected, analyzed, and displayed in a smooth, effective, and easily interpretable manner. This model would consist of goods that are distributed in a comparable way to standard commodities. Cloud services will include the virtual architecture for utility computing, which includes reporting, storage, analytics, visualization platforms, and client distribution. Businesses and customers would be able to access services on demand from everywhere thanks to the cost-based model that Cloud infrastructure provides [11-15].

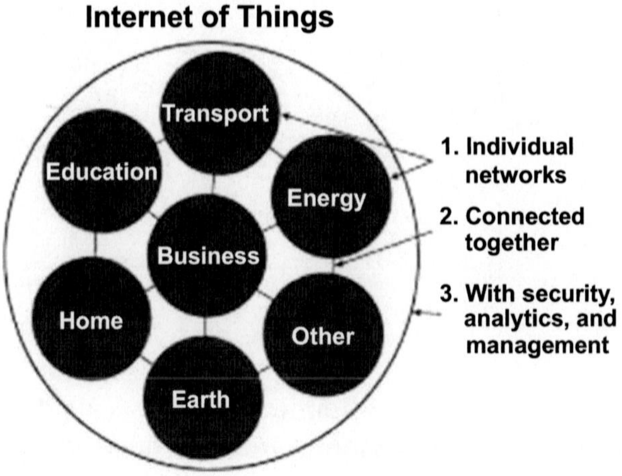

Fig. (1). Various applications in internet of things.

Internet of Things

IoT needs smart integration with current networks and context-aware computing utilizing network tools. The evolution toward universal knowledge and networking networks is already visible, with the growing presence of WiFi and 4G-LTE wireless Internet connectivity. However, in order for the Internet of Things vision to succeed, the computing criterion would need to expand past conventional mobile computing situations involving smart phones and portables, and into integrating ordinary existing devices and embedding information into our world. The Internet of Things requires a common knowledge of the condition of its consumers and their machines, software architectures and ubiquitous communication networks to store and communicate contextual knowledge to where it is important, and analytics tools in the Internet of Things that allow for autonomous and smart actions in order for technology to vanish from the user's consciousness. Smart integration and context-aware computing can be achieved with these three basic foundations in place. A transformative transformation of the modern Internet into a network of integrated objects that not only gathers data from the atmosphere (sensing) and communicates with the real universe (actuation/command/control), but also incorporates established Internet protocols to offer services for data transfer, analytics, software, and communications. IoT has grown out of its infancy and is on the brink of converting the existing static Internet into a truly developed.

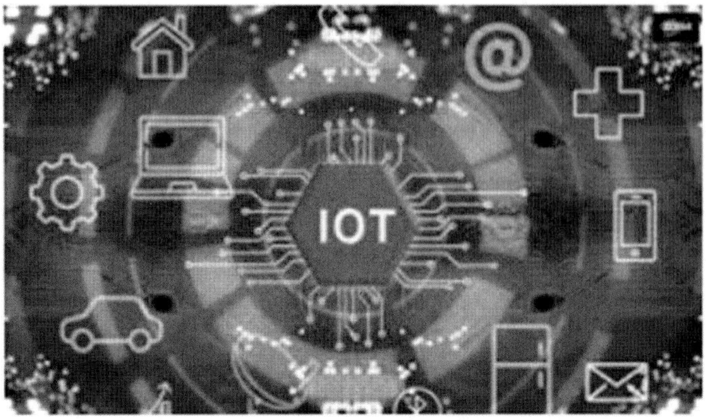

Fig. (2). Internet of things.

Future Internet, thanks to the proliferation of devices powered by accessible wireless technologies such as Bluetooth, radio frequency identification (RFID), Wi-Fi, and telephonic data networks, as well as embedded sensor and actuator nodes. The Internet revolution resulted in unparalleled levels of interconnection and speed between individuals. The interconnection of artifacts to build a smart world would be the next revolution. Their key incentive is to get their creative IoT goods and services to market as quickly as possible in order to achieve a competitive edge. As a result, many IoT devices and services are not built to be safe. Botnets and other forms of malicious malware are also being used to target the different weaknesses of IoT devices and services. This fact may pose a significant security danger because of the large number of IoT devices. For example, malicious software on devices can launch a major distributed denial of service (DDoS) assault against the target web site or information system. As a result, in the Internet of Things sector, protection is a critical research and technical subject. In addition, sensors produce a massive amount of data. Machine learning is the most popular approach for dealing with Big Data nowadays. The primary aim of our research is to provide an overview of machine learning techniques and methods used to improve IoT security, to classify the relevant state of the art research, and to identify possible future research ideas and challenges is shown in Fig. (**2**). The environment is rapidly changing from disconnected networks to pervasive Internet-enabled 'things' capable of communicating with one another and producing data that can be analysed to obtain useful knowledge. The Internet of Things, a massively integrated digital network system, would enhance everyone's existence, increase company growth, boost government performance, and so on. However, from the standpoint of protection and privacy, this modern reality (IoT) created on the Internet poses new problems. Because of the various requirements and networking stacks involved, traditional protection primitives cannot be explicitly extended to IoT technologies. Along with scalability and heterogeneity problems, resource-constrained systems like RFIDs and wireless sensor nodes make up a large part of IoT infrastructure. As a result, in such a complex setting, a scalable architecture capable of dealing with protection and privacy concerns is needed.

This paper provides an analysis of IoT protection and privacy problems, as well as current security strategies, as well as a list of open topics for potential study. The most significant inventions are those that vanish. They become indistinguishable from the structure of daily existence when they weave themselves through it. This Internet of Things idea has begun to transform our modern environment, including a common man's daily existence in society, a world in which machines of all shapes and sizes are produced with “smart” capabilities that enable them to connect and interact not only with other devices but also with humans, share data, make autonomous decisions, and perform useful tasks based on predetermined conditions. With its many implementations, the Internet of Things is now a well-known phenomenon across both horizontal and vertical industries. To illustrate how the Internet of Things could impact our everyday lives, consider the following scenario: You walk into the store and get a text message from your refrigerator.

Computing devices embedded in everyday items are connected through the Internet, allowing them to transmit and receive data. Nonetheless, modern IoT network technologies such as e-healthcare and transportation services have expanded this definition during the last decade. The Internet of Things arose from the integration of wireless technology, micro electromechanical systems (MEMS) advances, and digital electronics, resulting in small computers that can detect, calculate, and interact wirelessly. The connection or partnership between humans and machines is becoming increasingly important in the Internet of Things age, as machines get smarter and begin to do more human activities, and in this case, humans.

The next generation of computing will occur outside of the standard desktop setting. Many of the artifacts that accompany us would be linked in any way under the Internet of Things (IoT) model. This latest task, in which knowledge and communication networks are invisibly integrated in the world around us, would be met by RFID and sensor network technology. As a consequence, massive quantities of data are produced which must be collected, analyzed, and displayed in a smooth, effective, and easily interpretable manner. This model would consist of goods that are distributed in a comparable way to standard commodities. Cloud services will include the virtual architecture for utility computing, which includes reporting, storage, analytics, visualization platforms, and client distribution. Businesses and customers would be able to access services on demand from everywhere thanks to the cost-based model that Cloud infrastructure provides.

IoT needs smart integration with current networks and context-aware computing utilizing network tools. The evolution toward universal knowledge and networking networks is already visible, with the growing presence of WiFi and 4G-LTE wireless Internet connectivity. However, in order for the Internet of Things vision to succeed, the computing criterion would need to expand past conventional mobile computing situations involving smart phones and portables, and into integrating ordinary existing devices and embedding information into our world. The Internet of Things requires a common knowledge of the condition of its consumers and their machines, software architectures and ubiquitous communication networks to store and communicate contextual knowledge to where it is important, and analytics tools in the Internet of Things that allow for autonomous and smart actions in order for technology to vanish from the user's consciousness. Smart integration and context-aware computing can be achieved with these three basic foundations in place.

A transformative transformation of the modern Internet into a network of integrated objects that not only gathers data from the atmosphere (sensing) and communicates with the real universe (actuation/command/control), but also incorporates established Internet protocols to offer services for data transfer, analytics, software, and communications. IoT has grown out of its infancy and is on the brink of converting the existing static Internet into a truly developed Future Internet, thanks to the proliferation of devices powered by accessible wireless technologies such as Bluetooth, radio frequency identification (RFID), Wi-Fi, and telephonic data networks, as well as embedded sensor and actuator nodes. The Internet revolution resulted in unparalleled levels of interconnection and speed between individuals. The interconnection of artifacts to build a smart world would be the next revolution.

Their key incentive is to get their creative IoT goods and services to market as quickly as possible in order to achieve a competitive edge. As a result, many IoT devices and services are not built to be safe. Botnets and other forms of malicious malware are also being used to target the different weaknesses of IoT devices and services. This fact may pose a significant security danger because of the large number of IoT devices. For example, malicious software on devices can launch a major distributed denial of service (DDoS) assault against the target web site or information system. As a result, in the Internet of Things sector, protection is a critical research and technical subject. In addition, sensors produce a massive amount of data. Machine learning is the most popular approach for dealing with

Big Data nowadays. The target(s) are given to the machine learning algorithm, which then learns from the data which factors are critical in achieving the aim. This paper makes a significant impact by doing a comprehensive analysis of the current literature on machine learning for IoT defense. In the recent literature, there is no such systematic analysis. The above-mentioned paper did not address IoT protection. Our study's main goal is to provide a summary of machine learning strategies and methods used to enhance IoT security, classify applicable state-of-the-art research, and identify potential future research ideas and challenges. The biggest challenge today is figuring out how to coordinate, separate, and prioritize standardization efforts so that they can concentrate on the areas that bring the most value to customers, with the intention of speeding up rollout and achieving interoperable and stable IoT applications. Another significant obstacle is that IoT implementations must rely on specifications that have been established independently by various organisations or Technical Committees. Finally, interoperability (both communication and semantic) and certification of IoT software must be discussed.

VARIOUS SECTOR OF INTERNET OF THINGS

The Internet of Things is ushering in a modern age in computing technologies (IoT). IOT is a cloud-based "common global neural network" that links multiple devices. The Internet of Things (IoT) is a network of intelligently linked devices and networks made up of smart machines that interact and communicate with other machines, ecosystems, artifacts, and infrastructures, and RFID and sensor network technology will grow to face this new task. As a consequence, massive amounts of data are produced, collected, and analyzed into valuable activities that can "command and monitor" stuff to make our lives simpler and safer—while still reducing our environmental effects. Any organization, such as businesses and government agencies, requires current reports on individuals. In this respect, most businesses depend on blogs, newsletters, or bulletin boards. However, in most nations, internet connectivity is accessible to citizens on computers and mobile devices, making knowledge transfer far faster and less expensive through the internet (Fig. **3**).

The expression "Internet of Things" refers to network devices' capacity to sense and gather data from all over the world, and then distribute the data around the Internet, where it can be stored and used for a variety of fascinating purposes. The Internet of Things is made up of smart devices that connect and communicate with one another, as well as other machines, objects, systems, and infrastructures. Nowadays, everybody is linked to one another *via* a variety of contact channels. Whereas the internet is the most common mode of communication, we may argue that it is the internet that connects citizens.

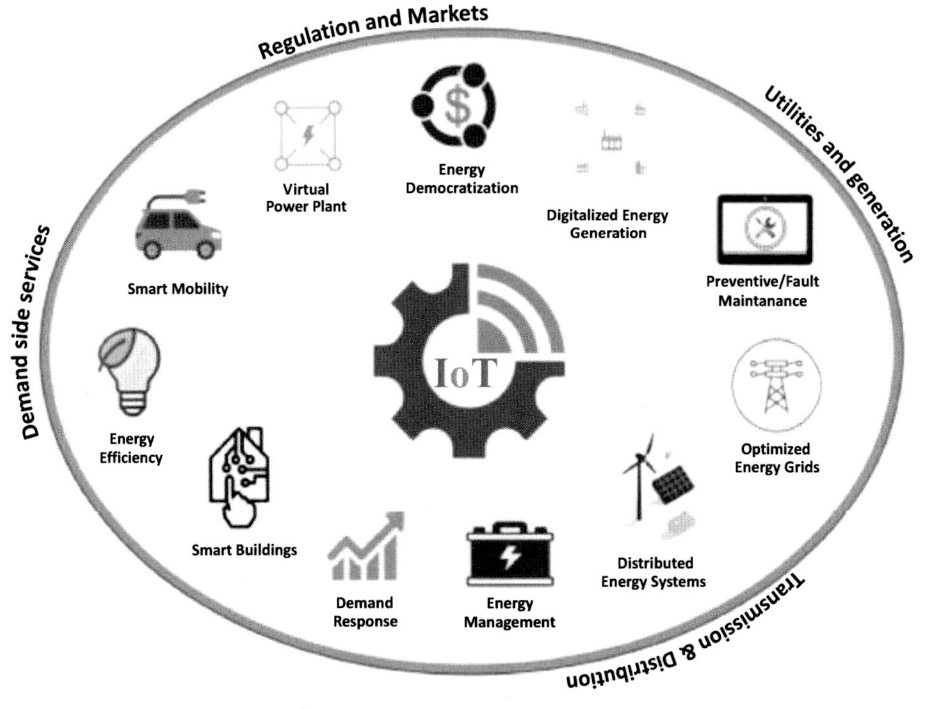

Fig. (3). Various sectors in internet of things.

The basic concept of the Internet of Things (IoT) has been around for nearly two decades, and it has drawn a lot of attention from academics and businesses because of its potential to improve our everyday lives and culture. When household appliances are linked to a network, they may collaborate to deliver the best service possible as a whole, rather than as a series of individually operating machines. This is useful for a variety of real-world technologies and utilities, such as building a smart home; for example, windows may be automatically closed when the air conditioner is switched on, or opened for oxygen when the gas oven is turned on. IoT systems may help human operations at a wider scale, such as a house or civilization, so the computers may collectively collaborate and function as a complete machine, which is particularly important for people with disabilities. These skills will then be used to create a whole class of services that make consumers' lives simpler. Not only does it collect data from the atmosphere (sensing) and communicate with the real universe (actuation/command/control), but it often makes use of established Internet protocols to include services such as data transfer, analytics, software, and communications. IoT has grown out of its infancy and is on the brink of converting the existing static Internet into a truly developed Future Internet, thanks to the proliferation of devices powered by accessible wireless technologies such as Bluetooth, radio frequency identification (RFID), Wi-Fi, and telephonic data networks, as well as embedded sensor and actuator nodes. The Internet revolution resulted in unparalleled levels of interconnection and speed between individuals. The interconnection of artifacts to build a smart world would be the next revolution. Nowadays, an information desk is needed at any railway station, shopping center, and college to provide information about the train schedule, promotional deals, and important notices. From the standpoint of an educational institution, the issue is that it necessitates certain workers who are committed to the task and who must be up to date with the institute and current events. The second issue is that in order to obtain details from the institute's information desk, an individual must first enter the institute. The solution is to utilize technology to make it accountable for answering all of the people's questions. Cell phones are the perfect option since they are accessible to nearly anyone and can be connected to the internet to download the most up-to-date material. In the event that the information is not changed through the internet, we must contact the customer care center for assistance. Some writers created a computer with all of the details contained in its database; if anyone requires information, they would use the device to obtain related information from it. In order for this to succeed, the system must be accessible to any person who requires assistance or encouragement. Students of educational establishments can be present in every area of the campus and may overlook vital information such as class rescheduling, for example. Furthermore, since students or clients might not be willing to walk through such notice boards on a daily basis, they might not be aware of crucial facts in order for it to be helpful to them. IoT enablement technologies include:

- The internet of things is enabled by three kinds of technologies: near-field networking, radio frequency identification (RFID), and cloud computing.

- RFID was the leading technology in the 2000s.

NFC became dominant within a few years (NFC). During the early 2010s, NFC became common in mobile phones, with applications such as reading NFC tags and gaining access to public transportation. This method is employed for low-cost labeling. Image-processing methods are used by phone cameras to decipher QR codes. In fact, QR advertising campaigns generate fewer buzz because consumers would use another app to interpret QR codes. This is a very new method. BLE hardware is used in all newly released smartphones. BLE tags will announce their existence at a low enough power level that they can run for up to a year on a lithium coin cell battery.

The Internet of Things (IoT) has the potential to significantly improve people's quality of life and business efficiency. The Internet of Things has the potential to enable extensions and improvements to fundamental services in transportation, logistics, defense, utilities, schooling, healthcare, and other fields, while also creating a new environment for application growth, thanks to a broadly dispersed, locally intelligent network of smart devices. To bring the industry beyond the early stages of business growth and into maturity, a concerted effort is needed, motivated by a shared awareness of the unique value of the potential. In terms of content delivery, company and charging structures, technologies needed to provide IoT services, and the different demands these services would pose on mobile networks, this industry has distinct characteristics. Connecting such smart devices (nodes) to the internet has begun as well, but at a slower rate. The parts of the technological puzzle are falling together faster than other people think to handle the Internet of Things. The Internet of Things could affect every part of our lives in less than a decade, much like the Internet phenomenon did not long ago and spread like wildfire. We've arrived at a point in life when nearly everybody has access to the Internet. The evolution in Internet technology has taken on a different form, allowing everything on the globe to communicate with one another, and this technology is known as IoT (Internet of Things). It's a massive phenomenon that's always changing, and the possibilities in IoT are endless. The number of people using the internet and the number of devices with internet access is growing.

With the Internet of Things (IoT) increasingly emerging as the next step of the Internet's development, it's more important than ever to consider the different possible domains for IoT implementations, as well as the study problems that come with them. IoT is set to penetrate almost any area of everyday life, from smart communities to health care, smart agriculture, logistics and shopping, and also smart living and smart ecosystems. Despite the fact that new IoT supporting solutions have vastly advanced in recent years, there are still a slew of issues that need to be addressed. Many research problems are bound to emerge since the IoT paradigm is based on heterogeneous technology. IoT is a significant research subject for studies in numerous relevant fields such as information technology and computer science since it is too broad and influences almost every aspect of our lives. As a result, the Internet of Things is opening the way for different types of analysis to be conducted. This paper addresses potential applications and technical issues as well as the latest progress of IoT technology.

The Internet is a networking network that links people to knowledge, while the Internet of Things (IoT) is a network of uniquely addressable physical objects with varying degrees of encoding, sensing, and actuation capabilities that share the capacity to interoperate and interact using the Internet as their common medium. As a result, the Internet of Things' primary goal is to enable artifacts to communicate with other objects, as well as individuals, at any time and from any place, *via* any network, route, or service. The Internet of Things (IoT) is increasingly being recognized as the next step in the development of the Internet. Ordinary computers would be able to link to the internet and accomplish a variety of objectives thanks to the Internet of Things. The internet has evolved from a mere network of machines to a network of numerous devices, and the internet of things (IoT) acts as a network of various "connected" devices, a network of networks. Smartphones, trucks, industrial systems, cameras, toys, buildings, home appliances, industrial systems, and a plethora of other gadgets will now all exchange data through the Internet. These instruments may perform smart reorganizations, tracing, tracking, control, real-time monitoring, and process management regardless of their size or purpose. There has been a significant increase in the number of Internet-capable smartphones in recent years. Even if the consumer electronics industry has seen the most important commercial impact, namely the mobile boom and interest in wearable technologies (watches, headphones, *etc.*), linking people has become merely a fragment of a larger trend towards the integration of the digital and physical worlds.

With all of this in mind, the Internet of Things (IoT) is predicted to continue to grow in terms of the amount of gadgets and functions it will support. This is shown by the uncertainty in the term "stuff," which allows defining the IoT's ever-expanding boundaries challenging. As market success begins to emerge, the Internet of Things (IoT) continues to have an almost unlimited supply of resources, not just in industry but also in science. As a result, the understudy discusses the different possible fields for IoT domain implementations as well as the analysis problems that come with them. The Internet of Things (IoT) allows anybody, at any time and in any location, to link to something, at any time and in any location. Through technological advancements, we are getting closer to a world in which all and all is linked. The Internet of Things (IoT) is regarded as the Internet's potential measurement, as it enables machine-to-machine (M2M) learning. The core concept behind the Internet of Things is to enable autonomous and safe data sharing and connection between real-world devices and applications. The Internet of Things (IoT) connects the physical and virtual worlds. The number of devices connecting to the Internet is rapidly growing. Personal computers, smartphones, tablets, mobile phones, PDAs, and other hand-held embedded devices are among these devices. Most mobile devices include a variety of sensors and actuators that can hear, compute, make intelligent decisions, and send valuable information across the Internet. The use of a network of such instruments with various sensors will result in a plethora of incredible applications and services that can provide tremendous personal, technical, and economic benefits. Items, sensing networks, networking platforms, computing and processing units that can be stored in the cloud, and decision-making and action-invoking systems make up the Internet of Things. The objects have some distinguishing characteristics, are easily recognizable, and can be accessed through the Internet. This physical items include Radio-Frequency Identification (RFID) tags or other identification barcodes that smart sensor sensors can detect. The sensors send object-specific data to the computational and processing device through the Internet. Smart services may be built using a variety of various sensors. The compilation outcome is then sent to the decision-making and action-invoking method, which decides which automatic action should be taken.

This paper looks at current development developments, IoT design in general, IoT defining characteristics, and potential future implementations. The Internet of Things (IoT) is a hot research subject that is gaining traction in education, business, and government. Many European and American organisations, as well as multinational corporations, are working on IoT design and production in order to provide a variety of valuable and efficient digital services. The Internet of Things faces numerous challenges in its implementation, especially in the areas of protection, regulation, and standardization, all of which are discussed in this article. In recent years, two rapidly changing technological subjects have been the Internet of Things (IoT) and Big Data. Big Data and the Internet of Things (IoT) go hand in hand. The IoT's key concept is that almost any entity or computer will have an IP address and will be connected to one another. With the assumption that trillions of machines would be connected and producing vast amounts of data, the reliability of data collection mechanisms would be tested. A wide range of organized and unstructured data, as well as a wide range of data models and query languages, as well as a wide range of data sources and veracity. This study paper discusses the problems of IoT for Big Data, including the criteria, technology utilized, data protection concerns, and other topics. IoT has been so relevant in our everyday lives that it would have a significant effect in the immediate future. For example, solutions for traffic flow can be delivered immediately, as well as reminders regarding car maintenance and energy conservation. Sensors can diagnose pending maintenance problems and will also prioritize maintenance team schedules for repair equipment. Data processing tools can make it easier for metropolitan and cosmopolitan communities to handle traffic, garbage, emission regulation, law enforcement, and other major functions effectively. Taking things a step forward, connected devices will assist individuals such as receiving a message from the refrigerator telling you to shop for food when the vegetable tray is bare, and the home protection system allowing you to unlock the door for any visitors *via* connected devices (IoT). The volume of data produced must be immense, given the huge increase in the number of devices every day. This is where Big Data and IoT come together. Big Data is in charge of managing the massive amounts of data produced by its technology. Big data and the Internet of

Things (IoT) are two important topics in commercial, manufacturing, and other applications. The term "Internet of Things" was coined around a decade ago to describe a world of computers or gadgets connecting to the Internet that capture, store, and process vast amounts of big data. Big data often applies to the study of this produced data in order to achieve meaningful outcomes. The gathering and processing of data relating to market transactions in order to discover who and when people purchase has been the driving force behind IoT and big data (Fig. **4**).

Big data storage must be able to manage extremely large volumes of data and provide constant juggling to keep up with growth, as well as provide the input/output operations per second (IOPS) needed to provide data to analytics software. Since the data is in various types and formats, a datacenter for storing it must be able to accommodate the load in various forms. Obviously, the Internet of Things has a strong effect on large data storage technology (Table **1**). IoT data collection Filtering redundant data is a must in Big Data, making it a difficult challenge. The data must then be sent over a network to a data center and stored. Many businesses have begun to use Platform as a Service (PaaS) to manage their IT technology. It aids in the creation and execution of web applications. Big data can be handled effectively in this manner without the need for specialized software.

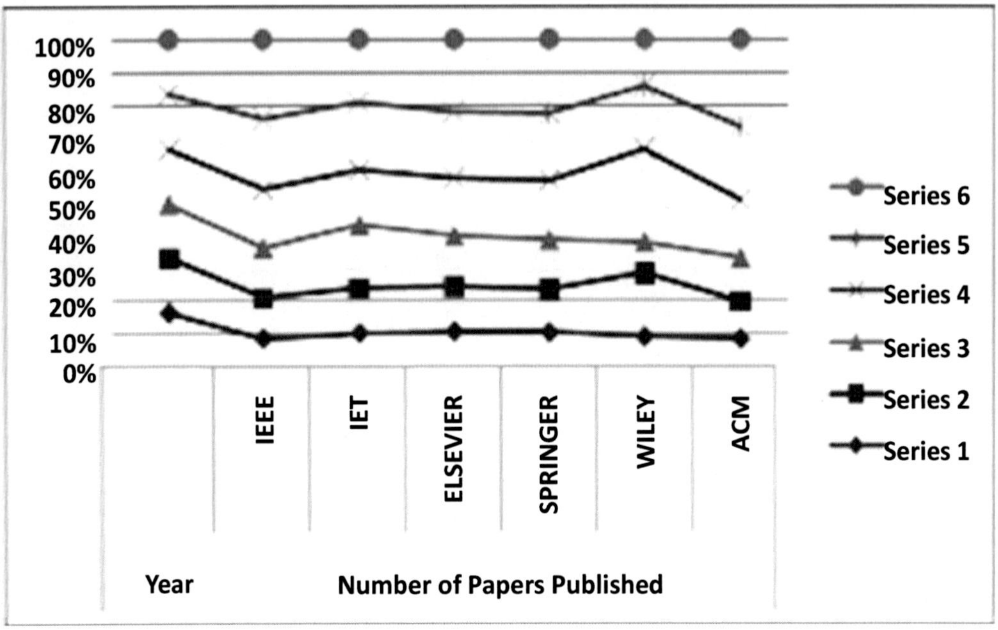

Fig. (4). Number of papers published in 2015-2020.

Table 1. Number of papers published in 2015-2020.

Year	Number of Papers Published					
	IEEE	IET	ELSEVIER	SPRINGER	WILEY	ACM
2015	15	22	25	50	10	20
2016	20	28	30	60	20	25
2017	25	40	35	70	10	30
2018	30	35	40	85	30	40
2019	35	42	45	95	20	50
2020	40	40	50	105	15	60

CONCLUSION

The paper gives a short overview of this widely used technology. We have joined a modern era of technology that has recently gained popularity; the technology's name is IoT, which stands for "Internet of Things." The Internet of Things (IoT) is also regarded as the Internet of All. The Internet of Things is made up of web-enabled devices that can interpret, receive, transmit, and react to data collected from the world by the use of highly functional sensors, communication hardware, network connections, and processors. The key goal of the Internet of Things is to transform real-world devices into intelligent abstract objects, making people's lives even simpler and easier. As we've noticed, contact is either human-human or human-device, but machine-machine communication did not exist prior to the advent of the Internet of Things. Because of the Internet of Things, this kind of contact (M2M) is feasible. The Internet boom, laptops, and other examples of the IoT's first step can be found. The Internet, also known as the cloud, is a worldwide system of interconnected networks that utilizes the TCP/IP (Transmission Control Protocol/Internet Protocol) protocol suite. The aim of this paper is to provide a broad overview of the well-known technological Internet of Things.

CONSENT FOR PUBLICATION

Not applicable.

CONFLICT OF INTEREST

The author declares no conflict of interest, financial or otherwise.

ACKNOWLEDGEMENT

Declared none.

REFERENCES

[1] Somayya Madakam, Ramaswamy R., and Siddharth Tripathi, "Internet of Things (IoT): A Literature Review",

[2] Emmanouil Vasilomanolakis, Jorg Daubert, Manisha Luthra, Vangelis Gazis, Alex Wiesmaie, and Panayotis Kikiras, *On the Security and Privacy of Internet of Things Architectures and Systems,* 2015. [http://dx.doi.org/10.1109/SIOT.2015.9]

[3] H. Shafagh, "Leveraging Public-keybased Authentication for the Internet of Things", *Master Thesis, RWTH Aachen University, Germany.,* 2013.

[4] R. Bonetto, N. Bui, V. Lakkundi, A. Olivereau, A. Serbanati, and M. Rossi, *Secure communication for smart IoT objects: Protocol stacks, use cases and practical examples*, 2012. http://dx.doi. Org /10.1109/WoWMoM.2012.626379010.1109/WoWMoM.2012.6263790

[5] C.D. Tuen, "Security in Internet of Things Systems", *Master Thesis Norwegian University of Science and Technology,* 2015.

[6] L. Coetzee, and J. Eksteen, "The Internet of Things-promise for the future? An introduction", In: *IST-Africa Conference Proceedings.* IEEE IEEE., 2011, 2011, pp. 1-9.

[7] Hongming Cai, Boyi Xu, Cheng Xie, Shaojun Qin, Lihong Jiang, and L. Jiang, Li Da Xu, "IoT-based configurable information service platform for product lifecycle management", *IEEE Trans. Industr. Inform.,* vol. 10, no. 2, pp. 1558-1567, 2014. [http://dx.doi.org/10.1109/TII.2014.2306391]

[8] R. Khan, S.U. Khan, R. Zaheer, and S. Khan, "Future internet: the internet of things architecture, possible applications and key challenges", In: *Frontiers of Information Technology (FIT),International Conference.* IEEE, 2012, 2012, pp. 257-260. [http://dx.doi.org/10.1109/FIT.2012.53]

[9] Y. Liu, and G. Zhou, "Key technologies and applications of internet of things", In: *Intelligent Computation Technology and Automation (ICICTA).* IEEE., 2012, pp. 197-200. [http://dx.doi.org/10.1109/ICICTA.2012.56]

[10] A.R. Sadeghi, C. Wachsmann, and M. Waidner, "Security and privacy challenges in industrial internet of things", In: *Proceedings of the 52nd annual design automation conference* ACM., 2015, p. 54. [http://dx.doi.org/10.1145/2744769.2747942]

[11] D.M. Blei, B.B. Edu, A.Y. Ng, A.S. Edu, M.I. Jordan, and J.B. Edu, "Latent Dirichlet Allocation", *CrossRef Listing of Deleted DOIs,* vol. 1, pp. 993-1022, 2000.

[12] P. Cisar, and S.M. Cisar, "General vulnerability aspects of Internet of Things", In: *International Symposium on Computational Intelligence and Informatics, Proceedings.* IEEE, 2016, pp. 117-121.

[13] G.A. Fink, D.V. Zarzhitsky, T.E. Carroll, and E.D. Farquhar, "Security and privacy grand challenges for the Internet of Things", In: *International Conference on Collaboration Technologies and Systems (CTS)* IEEE, 2015, pp. 27-34. [http://dx.doi.org/10.1109/CTS.2015.7210391]

[14] Gartner Inc, Gartner Says 6.4 Billion Connected, "Things", Will Be in Use in 2016,Up 30 Percent From 2015, 2016. http://www.gartner.com/newsroom/id/3165317

[15] Global Standards Initiative, Internet of Things Global Standards Initiative. http://www.itu.int/en /ITUT/ gsi/iot/Pages/default.aspx

CHAPTER 7

Secure Medical Data Transmission In Mobile Health Care System Using Medical Image Watermarking Techniques

B. Santhi[1] and **S. Priya**[1,*]

[1] *School of Computing, SASTRA Deemed to be University, Thanjavur, Tamilnadu, India*

Abstract: Medical information is maintained in a digital format, like scanned images along with patient information. In the mobile health care system, digitized medical information is transmitted to remote specialists for diagnosis purposes. The remote specialists verify the patient medical information using mobile or other devices and suggest the treatment. During medical data transmission, through unsecured media, there is a chance to modify the medical data by the attacker. It leads to the wrong diagnosis and affects the patient's entire life. So there is a need for secure medical data transmission in mobile healthcare to protect medical information from unauthorized users or intruders. The medical image watermarking technique is required to protect medical information in mobile healthcare. To withstand various medical image watermarking attacks, this chapter discusses two different types of robust medical image watermarking techniques in mobile healthcare. First, an intelligent-based medical image watermarking technique is discussed to protect the medical data in a secured manner during the electronic patient information embedding part. After embedding the patient information in the medical image, the generated watermarked medical image looks like an original medical image. So the attacker knows the visual existence of the medical data during its transmission. To avoid this, the second technique, *i.e.,* the visual medical image encryption technique, is discussed. The mobile healthcare system uses the intelligent medical image watermarking technique and visual medical image encryption for the secure transmission of medical information.

Keywords: Genetic algorithm, Image encryption, Medical image watermarking, Singular value decomposition, Visual image encryption.

INTRODUCTION

In the conventional medical system, the patient should be present physically, and the treatment is a very long time process. However, using the recent development

* **Corresponding author S. Priya:** School of Computing, SASTRA Deemed to be University, Thanjavur, Tamilnadu, India; Tel: 9952687066; E-mail: priya@ict.sastra.edu

Sivakumar R., Dimiter Velev, Basim Alhadidi, S. Vidhya, Sheeja V. Francis and B. Prabadevi (Eds.)

of Information and Communication Technology (ICT), an effective medical system is provided at a distance. Nowadays, a mobile health care system has been introduced to make the health care system effective, quick, and easy to access. With the prompt advancement in telecommunication and medicine, in the mobile health care system, the medical images are transmitted to the remote specialists along with the Electronic Patient Record (EPR) for diagnosis purposes. On the receiver side, the remote specialist uses this transmitted medical data for diagnosis purposes using mobile or other devices. It makes it easier to access. Due to this easy access, the mobile health care system compromises medical data security. Fig. (**1**) shows the mobile-based robust medical image watermarking technique.

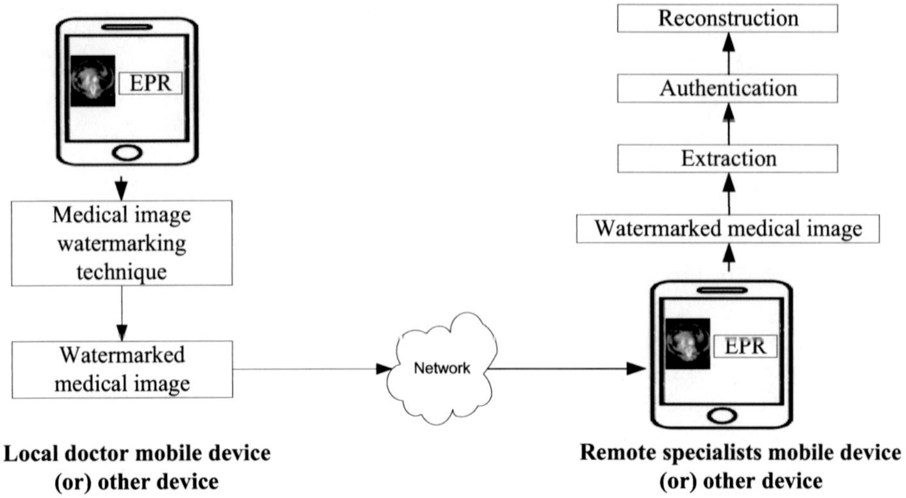

Fig. (1). Medical image watermarking in the mobile healthcare system.

So, one of the main challenging criteria in the mobile health care system is secure medical data transmission in open media. It is achieved by medical image watermarking techniques [1, 2]. In this technique, the electronic patient information is embedded within the medical image. Then the embedded watermarked medical image is transmitted to the remote specialist through mobile [3]. At the remote specialist side, the transmitted watermarked medical image is received and used for the diagnosis.

Image watermarking techniques are divided into different types based on the working domain (Spatial & Transform), Human Visual System characteristics (HVS), fragile- and robust-based [4, 5]. To transmit the medical image in a secured manner against various attacks, a transformed-based robust watermarking technique is required. So this chapter focus on robust medical image watermarking techniques in the mobile health care system.

Singular value decomposition and DWT are used to generate the robust medical image watermarking technique [4]. SHA-512 is used to generate the digital signature for the iris image. In the region of non-interest part, the watermark information (EPR, Digital signature, reference watermark) is embedded. It requires more time for hash value generation. For telemedicine [5], robust dual medical image watermarking is generated. Singular Value Decomposition (SVD) and Discrete Wavelet Transform (DWT) are used to increase the embedding capacity. Multiple watermarking techniques are proposed in the transform domain using DWT, DCT, and SVD [6].

Electronic patient information is embedded in the medical image using Gould and integer wavelet transform to increase security. However, its embedding capacity is low [7]. Therefore, an encryption-based watermarking technique is proposed in telemedicine. A chaotic-based fragile watermarking technique is proposed with a high payload in a cloud environment [8], but it does not withstand against robustness attack. Furthermore, a robust watermarking technique is proposed using spatial and transform domains [9]. Within the singular component, the watermark information is embedded. A spread spectrum-based medical image watermarking technique is also proposed [10].

In all the previous methods, the watermarked medical image is similar to the original medical image. So the attacker visually knows the medical image transmission. To avoid the visual existence, watermarking method image encryption technique is used. The image encryption output is similar to noisy data or modified data. It depicts that some secret information is present in an unreadable format. Therefore, to overcome the drawbacks of the existing methods, this chapter discusses the two types of security techniques for mobile healthcare systems. To increase the robustness of the medical image watermarking technique, the intelligent-based watermarking technique using a genetic algorithm is discussed, and to avoid the visual existence of the medical image watermarking technique, a visually meaningful image encryption technique is discussed.

Performance Measures

To evaluate the performance of the medical image watermarking techniques, the following metrics from Equations **1-5** are considered in this chapter. In all the metrics, the original medical image is referred to as the X, and the watermarked medical image is considered as X' with the pixel position as (u,v) and size as MXN.

Peak Signal to Noise Ratio (PSNR)

PSNR value is calculated to measure the quality of the original medical image compared to the watermarked medical image. For high PSNR value, high image quality is obtained.

$$PSNR = 10\log_{10}\left(\frac{255^2}{MSE}\right) \quad \textbf{(1)}$$

where MSE is the mean squared error between original and watermarked image, it is defined as,

$$MSE = \frac{\sum_{u=0}^{m-1}\sum_{v=0}^{n-1}\left(X(u,v)-\left(X'(u,v)\right)\right)^2}{mXn} \quad \textbf{(1a)}$$

Normalized Cross-Correlation (NCC)

Correlation between the two images is measured using NCC. If the two images are the same, the NCC value is otherwise 0.

$$NCC = \frac{\sum_{u=0}^{m-1}\sum_{v=0}^{n-1} X(u,v).X'(u,v)}{\sum_{u=0}^{m-1}\sum_{v=0}^{n-1} X'(u,v)^2} \quad \textbf{(2)}$$

Structural Similarity Index (SSIM)

Structural information degradation is measured by SSIM. SSIM value lies between 0 and 1.

$$SSIM = I(u,v).C(u,v).S(u,v), \quad \textbf{(3)}$$

where I is the luminance, C is the contrast, and S is the structural component between two images.

Number of Pixels Change Rate (NPCR)

This is used to measure the pixel changes in the original standard image (A) with its encrypted image (A'). If the NPCR value is low, then the difference is low. It means both A and A' are the same.

$$NPCR = \frac{\sum_{u,v} dif(u,v)}{MXN} X100\%, \tag{4}$$

where,

$$diff(u,v) = \begin{cases} o & if\ A(u,v) = A'(u,v)) \\ 1 & if\ A(u,v) \neq A'(u,v) \end{cases} \tag{4a}$$

Unified Average Changing Intensity (UACI)

UACI is used to calculate the average pixel intensity changes between the original and its ciphered image using Equation **10**.

$$UACI = \frac{1}{MXN} \sum_{i,j} \frac{A(u,v) - A'(u,v)}{255} \tag{5}$$

where MXN is the size of the image, A andA' are the original and its encrypted image, respectively. If the UACI value is low, then A and A' are the same.

INTELLIGENT BASED REVERSIBLE MEDICAL IMAGE WATERMARKING

For secure transmission of medical images, an intelligent-based robust medical image watermarking technique is proposed. Using Integer Wavelet Transform (IWT) and singular value decomposition (SVD), the medical image is decomposed. To withstand various attacks, in singular values of SVD, the EPR data are embedded, and watermarked medical image is generated.

Preliminaries

Integer Wavelet Transform (IWT)

In the existing transform-based robust watermarking techniques, DWT (Discrete Wavelet Transform) is used. It recovers the data with loss. In DWT, the integer values are converted into floating-point values, and secret data are embedded by modifying that values. So there is no guarantee for the exact recovery of that integer values at the receiver side. So no proper recovery of the medical information leads to a wrong diagnosis. To avoid this problem, an integer wavelet transform is used. IWT decomposes the image into four subparts. Then the EPR data is embedded within any subpart of the wavelet coefficient.

Singular Value Decomposition (SVD)

It divides the matrix into three independent components (two orthogonal matrices and one diagonal matrix) for analysis. All three components have different sizes. The following Equation **6** represents the SVD decomposition of the image (I) with MXN size. in which U and V^T represent the orthogonal matrices, D represents the diagonal matrix.

$$[UDV^T] = SVD(I)$$

$$UDV^T = \begin{bmatrix} u_{1,1} & u_{1,2} & \cdots & u_{1,M} \\ u_{2,1} & u_{2,2} & \cdots & u_{2,M} \\ \vdots & \vdots & \ddots & \vdots \\ u_{M,1} & u_{M,2} & \cdots & u_{M,M} \end{bmatrix} X \begin{bmatrix} D_{1,1} & 0 & \dots & 0 \\ 0 & D_{2,2} & \cdots & 0 \\ \vdots & \vdots & \ddots & \vdots \\ 0 & 0 & \cdots & D_{M,N} \end{bmatrix} X \begin{bmatrix} v_{1,1} & v_{1,2} & \cdots & u_{1,N} \\ v_{2,1} & v_{2,2} & \cdots & v_{2,N} \\ \vdots & \vdots & \ddots & \vdots \\ v_{N,1} & v_{N,2} & \dots & v_{N,N} \end{bmatrix}^T \quad \textbf{(6)}$$

Genetic Algorithm (GA)

The genetic algorithm was introduced with the base of evolutionary models. This is one of the important tools for selecting the optimum parameters. GA consists of five important operations such as random number generation, fitness function evolution, selection, cross-over, and mutation. The random number generated from the pseudo-random generator is considered as the initial population. The fitness function is used to evaluate the optimum parameters. The selection function selects the seed value. Cross-over operation selects parent string and divides it into two equal parts. Then combine the differential pair from the child strings. Mutation operation reverses or inverts the strings of bits. The mutation operation depends on the mutation rate.

Intelligent Based Medical Image Watermarking (IMW)

The medical image of size MxN is analyzed to embed the watermark. SVD is applied to the original medical image using Equations **7** and **8**. The singular component of the SVD is considered to embed the secret data.

$$I = IWT(M) \quad \textbf{(7)}$$

$$[PQR'] = SVD(I) \quad \textbf{(8)}$$

In Equations **7** and **8**, M is the original medical image, I is the wavelet transformed image, P and R' are orthogonal matrix, Q is the singular component of the matrix. The singular matrix is not get affected by the various attack. So the watermark is embedded in a singular matrix along with the scaling factor â (scaling is 0.5) using Equations **9** and **10**. After that, inverse SVD is applied to the embedded matrix. Then inverse IWT is obtained to generate a watermarked medical image (I_{wd}).

$$Q_w = Q + \beta \, . w \tag{9}$$

$$I_w = P . Q_w \, . R' \tag{10}$$

Then using GA, an intelligent based watermarking technique is generated. After the patient information is embedded in the medical image, various watermarking attacks are applied to the watermarked medical image (I_{wd}). Then the attacked medical image is transmitted to the receiver. At the receiver, from that image, secrete data are extracted. Then performance measures are calculated, and fitness function is applied. This process is repeated until the optimum parameter is selected to embed the watermark to withstand the various attack. Fig. (**2**) shows the proposed method. The fitness function is calculated using the following three performance metrics, such as PSNR, NC, and SSIM, by considering the following Equation **11**.

$$f_m = (PSNR_m + SSIM_m + NC_m) \tag{11}$$

The intelligent-based watermarking method is illustrated as follows:

1. Apply IWT and SVD to the original medical image.

2. Embed the watermark information (patient) within a singular component of the transformed image.

3. Apply attack on watermarked medical image.

4. Using the GA training process, the optimum parameter is obtained to withstand various attacks.

5. Until the optimum parameter is found, the GA training process is repeated.

6. Once the optimum parameter is obtained, the watermark information is embedded using that parameter to withstand the various attack.

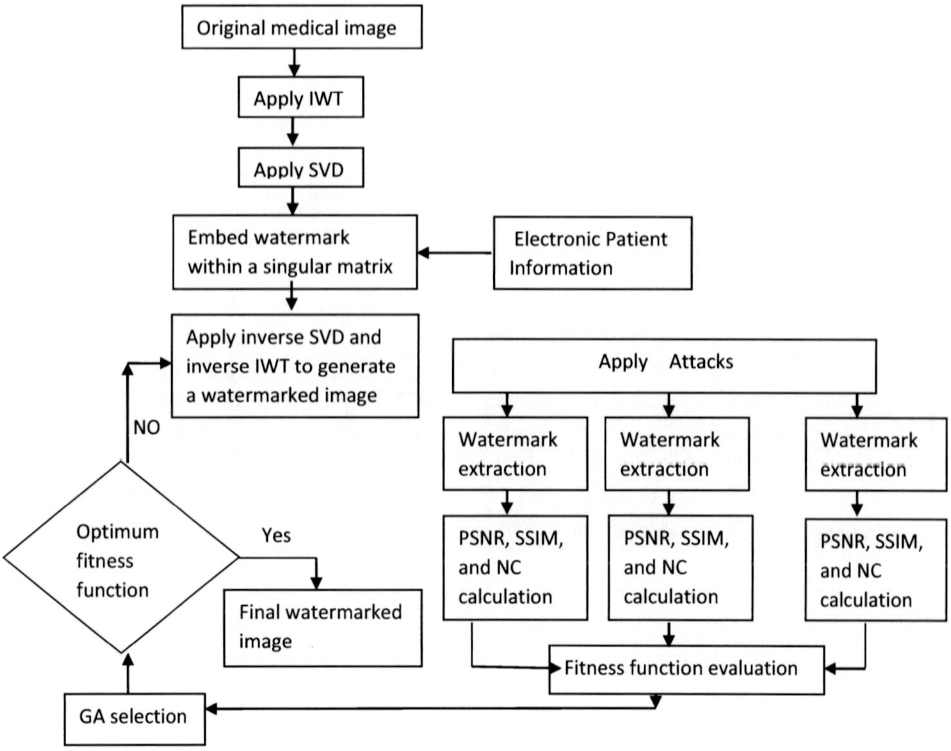

Fig. (2). Intelligent based medical image watermarking.

Watermark Extraction

The watermark information is extracted by reversing the watermark embedding process. IWT and SVD are applied to the watermarked medical image. From singular matrix, watermark information is extracted without any loss.

Experimental Results

The performance of the intelligent watermarking methods was evaluated using the online MAT Lab tool. Various medical images from ANBU hospital, Kumbakonam, Tamilnadu, and standard ordinary images of Lena and Barbara are considered. The medical image size is considered as 512X512. For the GA training process, 10 individuals are considered for each iteration. Scattered mutation function and stochastic uniform selection operation is taken from the GA toolbox. For mutation, the Gaussian function is considered.

The output images are shown in Fig. (**3**). It shows that visually the watermarked medical image is similar to the original medical image. Some geometric and signal processing attacks are considered to evaluate the robustness of the proposed method. The PSNR value for the various medical image is listed in Table **1**. The PSNR values are more than 35Db. Fig. (**4**) shows the NCC values by considering the various attacks. The NCC values for all the images are greater than 0.7, which is closer to 1. It shows that the proposed method withstands the various attacks. The watermark information was also retrieved without any loss.

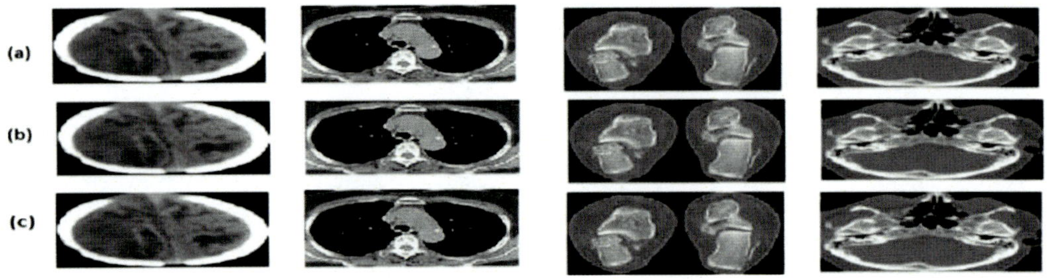

Fig. (3). Medical images (brain, chest, foot, face). **(a)** Original images **(b)** Watermarked images **(c)** Reconstructed images.

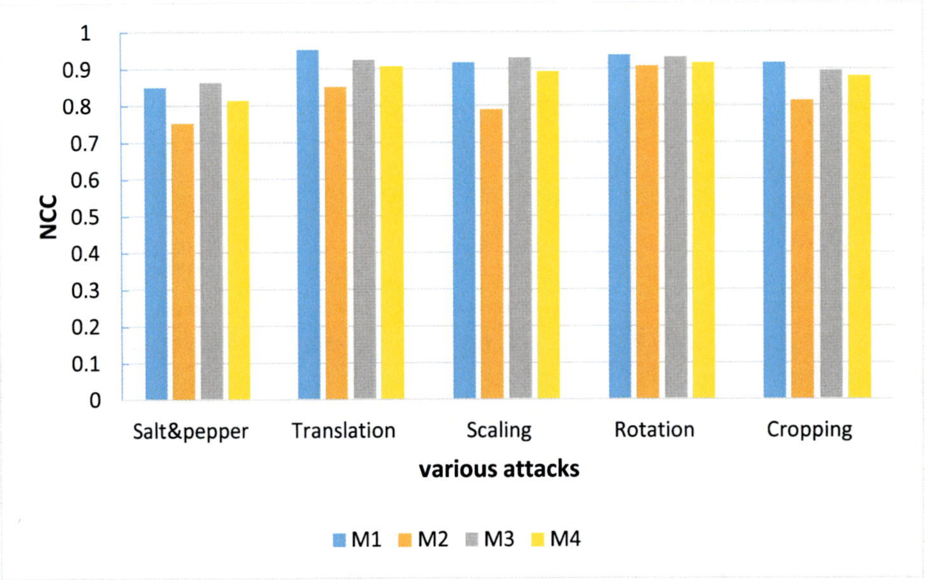

Fig. (4). NCC values for various medical images with attacks.

Table 1. PSNR (dB) values.

Types of Attacks	Various Medical Images			
	M1	M2	M3	M4
Salt & pepper	44.43	45.69	47.12	46.31
Translation	40.23	40.89	41.35	40.22
Scaling	43.21	39.89	39.13	41.34
Rotation	39.23	38.12	40.03	38.45

VISUALLY MEANINGFUL IMAGE ENCRYPTION (VMIE)

After the watermarked medical image is generated using the previous method, it is transmitted to the remote specialist. The watermarked medical image is visually similar to the original medical image. Then the attacker visually knows the transmission of the medical image. To avoid this, the image encryption technique is used to protect the medical image from attackers. Normal image encryption is used to transform the secret image into an encrypted image to withstand various cryptographic attacks. The normal encrypted image looks like a noise-based or texture-based image. Image encryption only protects the secret image, not its existence. The output noise or texture-based structure shows the existence of the secret image. Then, the attacker easily predicts some secrete information is transmitted in an unreadable format. So to avoid the visual existence of the watermarked medical image, visually meaningful image encryption is used [11 - 14]. That is, the watermarked medical image is encrypted as a significant encrypted image. It is explained below.

An ordinary standard image like Lena, baboon, peppers, *etc.,* is considered as the reference image. The reference image of size 2MX2N size is considered as the cover image (C). Apply IWT to reference cover image (C). The level of the wavelet decomposition depends on the user requirement. This chapter is considered the decomposition level as 2. For authentication purposes, the sender finger print's also taken into account along with the watermarked medical image. The fingerprint image is converted into a binary image format (B) and embedded within the LSB bit of the wavelet coefficient.

Then the watermarked image of size MXN is embedded within the coefficients of the wavelet subband using any one of the visual image encryption techniques [11 - 14]. The encrypted cypher image (C') visually looks like an ordinary image. So for the attackers, it is very tough to detect the transmitted medical image.

The VMIE is defined using the following Equation.

$$C' = E(W', C, B, n) \quad \textbf{(12)}$$

Where E is the encryption function, W' is the watermarked medical image, C is the reference image, n is the levels of IWT, and C' is the final encrypted image. The detailed structure of the VMIE is shown in Figs. (**5** and **6**). The proposed method algorithm is illustrated as follows.

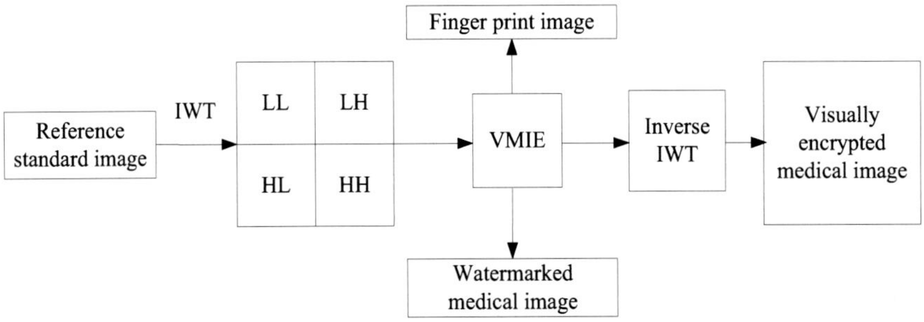

Fig. (5). VMIE Encryption at the sender side.

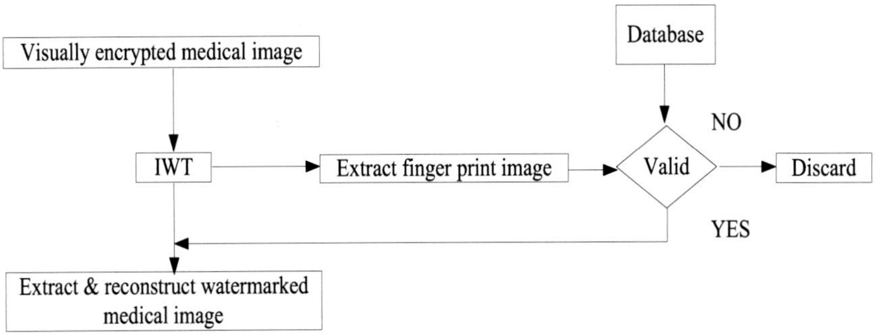

Fig. (6). VMIE decryption at the receiver side.

1. Consider an image with 2MX2N as a reference image (C).

2. Apply IWT to C to decompose the image into subbands.

3. Consider the binary format of the sender's signature.

4. Encrypt the watermarked medical image (O') with any of the wavelet subbands (LL, LH, HL, HH) of the reference image (C) using the existing visual image encryption.

5. Apply inverse IWT to generate a visually meaningful encrypted medical image (C').

Decryption and Authentication

At the receiver side, the encrypted medical image (C ‘) is divided into sub-bands using IWT. From the subband, the doctor's fingerprint image and watermarked medical image are extracted. The decryption process is shown in Fig. (**6**). The extracted fingerprint image is validated with the database image. If it is valid, then the extracted watermarked medical image is considered and reconstructed for further process. It is represented using the following Equation **13**.

$$(B, W') = D(C', n) \quad \textbf{(13)}$$

where C’ is the encrypted watermarked medical image, D is the decryption process, n is the levels of the wavelet decomposition, B is the extracted fingerprint binary image, and W’ is the extracted watermarked medical image.

Experimental Analysis

The proposed method is analyzed with various DICOM medical [15] images and standard images [11]. The original and its visually encrypted images are shown in Fig. (**3**). It shows that, visually, the encrypted images are similar to the original images. It says that the proposed method prevents the visual existence of the original image. It is impossible to differentiate the original and its encrypted image. Table **1** lists out the PSNR values of the various encrypted image. The values are greater than 30dB, so it is acceptable by the human visual system. The PSNR values of the extracted watermark compared with the original watermark are infinite. It proves that there is no data loss in the extracted data using the visual image encryption method. Fig. (**7**) shows the watermarked images before and after encryption, and both images are the same without any loss.

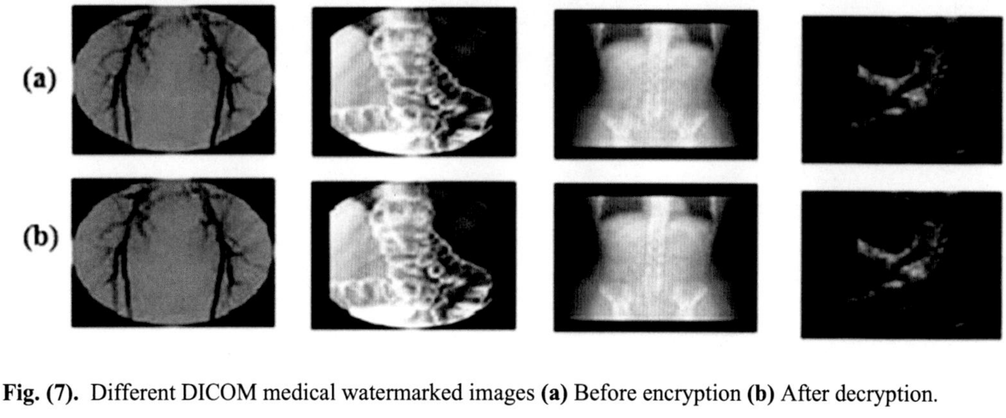

Fig. (7). Different DICOM medical watermarked images **(a)** Before encryption **(b)** After decryption.

Keyspace Analysis

The Integer wavelet transform is used for visual image encryption. Totally 37 wavelet filters are used, and the decomposition level depends on the user's level (n). So the keyspace for the proposed method is 37^n. It shows that the proposed method is not breakable using a brute force attack.

Histogram Attack

Histograms of the various watermarked and encrypted images are shown in Fig. (**8**). It shows that the histogram of the output ciphered (encrypted) image is different from the watermarked image histogram. And the Peppers image is used to encrypt the different watermarked medical images. But the histogram of all the Peppers cipher images is visually similar. For the attackers, it is very difficult to break the system to detect the watermarked medical image. Hence the proposed method withstands the histogram attacks.

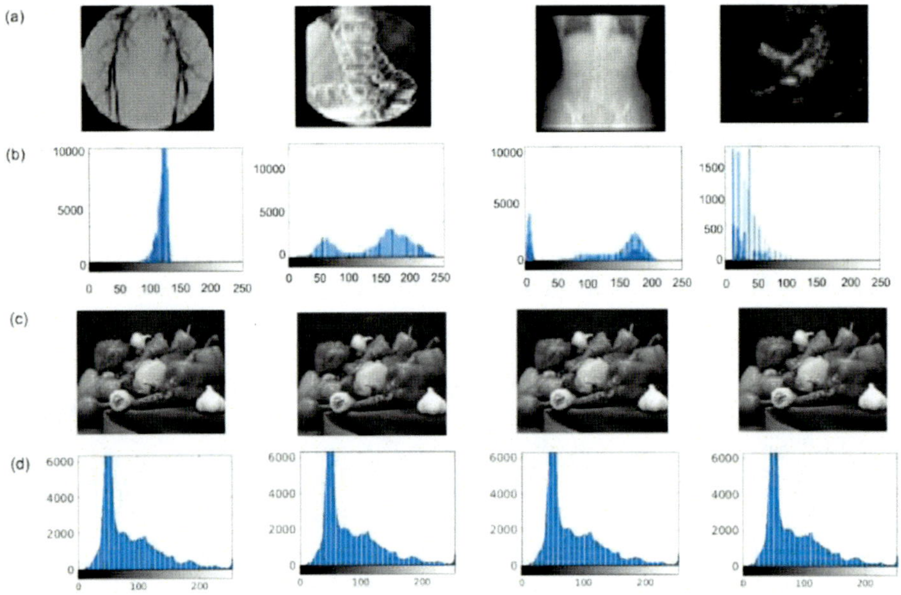

Fig. (8). Histogram (**a** and **b)** different watermarked medical images with its corresponding histogram (**c** and **d)** encrypted image with its corresponding histogram.

Differential Attack

This analysis is mainly used to measure the variations of the original image pixel values with the cypher image pixel value. NPCR (Number of Pixel Change Rate) and UACI (Unified Average Changing Intensity) are the two measures used to evaluate the differential attack. Fig. (**9**) shows the NPCR and UACI values for the various standard image. NPCR value is less than 60, and UACI value is closer to 0. It shows that the, visually the medical watermarked images are not identified by the attackers.

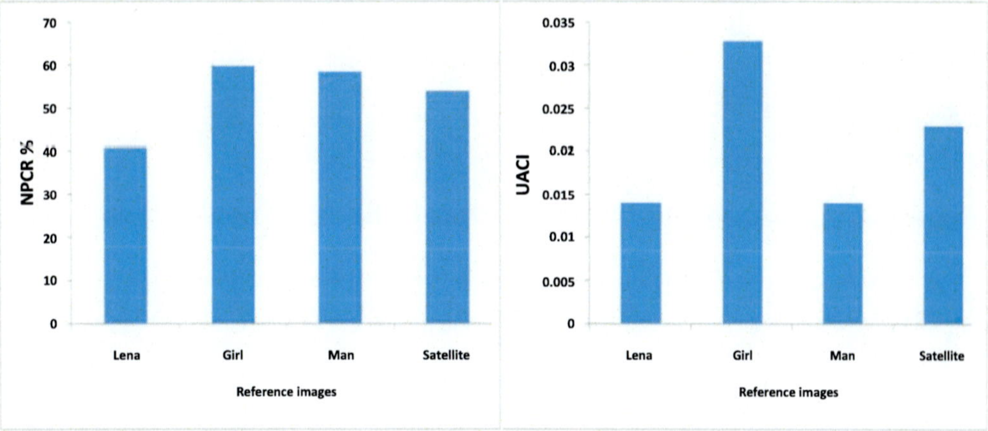

Fig. (9). NPCR and UACI values.

CONCLUSION

This chapter discusses two robust medical image watermarking techniques for secure medical data transmission in the mobile healthcare system. In the first method, an intelligent-based robust medical image watermarking technique is considered using a genetic algorithm. In this method, EPR data are embedded using IWT and SVD. The optimum parameter is obtained using a genetic algorithm. This robust intelligent based medical image watermarking technique withstands various geometric and signal processing attacks. In the second method, visual meaningful image encryption is discussed to overcome the visual attack. This method avoids the visual existence of the medical watermarked image by using the wavelet transform. It also provides the senders' authentication by embedding their fingerprint images along with the EPR. The performance measures show that the two robust medical image watermarking techniques provide secure medical data transmission in the mobile healthcare system.

CONSENT FOR PUBLICATION

Not applicable.

CONFLICT OF INTEREST

The author declares no conflict of interest, financial or otherwise.

ACKNOWLEDGEMENTS

The authors would like to thank ANBU hospital, Kumbakonam, Tamilnadu, India, for giving the original scanned medical image for this research work.

REFERENCES

[1] S.M. Mousavi, A. Naghsh, and S.A.R. Abu-Bakar, "Watermarking techniques used in medical images: a survey", *J. Digit. Imaging,* vol. 27, no. 6, pp. 714-729, 2014. [http://dx.doi.org/10.1007/s10278-014-9700-5] [PMID: 24871349]

[2] A.F. Qasim, and F. Meziane, *F and R. Aspin. "Digital watermarking Applicability for developing trust in medical imaging workflows state of the art review".* vol. 27. Comput. Sci. Rev, 2018, pp. 45-60.

[3] C.N. Gutierrez, G. Kakani, R.C. Verma, and T. Wang, Digital watermarking of medical images for mobile devices.*IE.* EE Int Conf on Sensor Networks, Ubiquitous, and Trustworthy Computing, 2010, pp. 421-425.

[4] R. Pandey, "Iris based secure NROI multiple eye image watermarking for teleophthalmology", *Multimed Tools Appl.,* vol. 75, no. 22, pp. 14381-14397, .

[5] A.K. Singh, B. Kumar, M. Dave, and A. Mohan, "Robust and imperceptible dual watermarking for telemedicine applications", *Wirel. Pers. Commun.,* vol. 80, no. 4, pp. 1415-1433, 2015. [http://dx.doi.org/10.1007/s11277-014-2091-6]

[6] A.K. Singh, M. Dave, and A. Mohan, "Hybrid technique for robust and imperceptible multiple watermarking using medical images", *Multimedia Tools Appl.,* vol. 75, no. 14, pp. 8381-8401, 2016. [http://dx.doi.org/10.1007/s11042-015-2754-7]

[7] P. Selvam, S. Balachandran, S.P. Iyer, and R. Jayabal, *Hybrid transform-based reversible watermarking technique for medical images in telemedicine applications.* vol. 145. Optik, 2017, pp. 655-671.

[8] X. Cao, Z. Fu, and X. Sun, "A privacy-preserving outsourcing data storage scheme with fragile digital watermarking-based data auditing", *J. Electr. Comput. Eng.,* vol. 2016, pp. 1-7, 2016. [http://dx.doi.org/10.1155/2016/3219042]

[9] I.A. Ansari, and M. Pant, *M. "Multipurpose image watermarking in the domain of DWT based on SVD and ABC".* vol. 94. Pattern Recognit. Lett, 2017, pp. 228-236.

[10] A.K. Singh, B. Kumar, M. Dave, and A. Mohan, "Multiple watermarking on medical images using selective discrete wavelet transform coefficients", *J. Med. Imaging Health Inform.,* vol. 5, no. 3, pp. 607-614, 2015. [http://dx.doi.org/10.1166/jmihi.2015.1432]

[11] R. Ponuma, R. Amutha, S. Aparna, and G. Gopal, "Visually meaningful image encryption using data hiding and chaotic compressive sensing", *Multimedia Tools Appl.,* vol. 78, no. 18, pp. 25707-25729, 2019. [http://dx.doi.org/10.1007/s11042-019-07808-6]

[12] Y.G. Yang, B.P. Wang, Y.L. Yang, Y.H. Zhou, W.M. Shi, and X. Liao, *Visually meaningful image encryption based on universal embedding model.* vol. 562. Inf. Sci, 2021, pp. 304-324.

[13] S. Arunkumar, V. Subramaniyaswamy, R. Devika, and R. Logesh, "Generating visually meaningful encrypted image using image splitting technique", *J. Mech. Eng Technol.,* vol. 8, no. 8, pp. 368-391, 2017.

[14] S. Priya, and B. Santhi, "A novel visual medical image encryption for the secure transmission of authenticated watermarked medical images", *Mob. Netw. Appl.,* pp. 1-8, 2019.

[15] DICOM sample image sets [Online]. Available, http//www.barre.nom.fr/medical/samples

CHAPTER 8

Smartphone-Based Real-Time Monitoring and Forecasting of Drinking Water Quality using LSTM and GRU in IoT Environment

V. Murugan[1,*], J. Jeba Emilyn[2] and M. Prabu[3]

[1] *Trichy Engineering College, Trichy-621132, Tamil Nadu, India*

[2] *Sona College of Technology, Salem-636005, Tamil Nadu, India*

[3] *National Institute of Technology Calicut, Kozhikode -673601, Kerala, India*

Abstract: Water quality plays an important role in human health. Contamination of drinking water resources causes waterborne diseases like diarrhoea and even some deadly diseases like cancer, kidney problems, *etc.* The mortality rate of waterborne diseases is increasing every day and most school children get affected to a great extent. Real-time monitoring of water quality of drinking water is a tedious process and most of the existing systems are not automated and can work only with human intervention. The proposed system makes use of the Internet of Things (IoT) for measuring water quality parameters and recurrent neural networks for analysing the data. An IoT kit using raspberry pi is developed and connected with a GPS module and proper sensors for measuring pH, temperature, nitrate, turbidity, and dissolved oxygen. The measured water quality data can be sent directly from raspberry pi to the database server or through the mobile application by QR code scanning. Recurrent Neural Network algorithms namely Long Short-Term Memory (LSTM) and Gated Recurrent Unit (GRU) are used for forecasting water quality. Results show that analysis made using GRU is much faster than LSTM, whereas prediction of LSTM is slightly more accurate than GRU. The data is categorized as poor, moderate, or good for drinking and it can be accessed using smartphones through mobile application. In general, the proposed system produces accurate results and can be implemented in schools and other drinking water resources.

Keywords: Gated Recurrent Unit, Internet of Things, Long Short-Term Memory, Recurrent Neural Networks, Water Quality Parameters.

* **Corresponding author V. Muruga:** Trichy Engineering College, Konalai, Trichy-621132, Tamil Nadu, India; Tel: 9698814584; E-mail: muruganv84@gmail.com

Sivakumar R., Dimiter Velev, Basim Alhadidi, S. Vidhya, Sheeja V. Francis and B. Prabadevi (Eds.)

INTRODUCTION

In most parts of the world,especially in India, groundwater is used for drinking. Around one and half million people of the world population rely upon groundwater for drinking purposes [1]. With an increase in world population, high industrialization, use of excessive fertilizers, reduction in rainfall, *etc.*, the quality of groundwater is deteriorating [2, 3, 4]. Rivers, dams, and ponds are all sources of surface water, meeting the need for drinking water to some extent. Due to the lack of surface water, drinking water is provided to people through transportation. Drinking water either groundwater or surface water results in diseases caused by water-borne agents due to inadequate quality of water.

The water quality is governed by physical and chemical properties of water such as temperature, dissolved oxygen, nitrate content, turbidity, *etc.* Turbidity is a term that checks the concentration of extraneous particles in water. Drinking water with a large quantity of dissolved oxygen is good, and it also makes the water taste better. Groundwater and surface water are contaminated by nitrate due to the excessive use of nitrogen fertilizers, and the consumption of high amounts of nitrate adversely affects health. Excess nitrate consumption can lead to cardiovascular disease, stomach cancer, lung disease, *etc.*

pH of drinking water is a measure of charged particles in drinking water. The pH of good drinking water should lie between 6.5 – 7.5. A low value of pH indicates acidic properties and a higher value of pH indicates alkaline properties. Both too much acidity and alkalinity are not good for human health. Drinking water contaminated with nitrate has severe impacts on human health.

Human body parts that are prone to cancer due to nitrate contamination are the urinary bladder, brain, rectum, kidney, pancreas, breast, ovary, and stomach [5 - 12]. Overconsumption of nitrate by pregnant women may lead to premature births, birth defects of the abdominal wall, low birth weight, gastroschises, *etc.* in newborns [13 - 16].

Several other diseases related to the central nervous system and thyroid have a close association with nitrate ingestion. Several recent studies show that gastrointestinal (GI) illness that occurred in the US is a water-borne disease and has proximity to turbidity of water [17]. Alkaline drinking having higher pH doesn’t cause adverse health effects and even can be used in the treatment of reflux disease [18] whereas, on the other hand, acidic drinking water which has low pH can be a root cause of diseases like diarrhoea, abdominal pain, organ damage, nausea, and vomiting. Acidity in water is mainly due to toxic metals that are mixed with water [19].

E. coli (Escherichia coli) bacteria that live in human or some animal intestines is transmitted to surface water through human faecal material.

Although most *E. coli* are not dangerous, some of them are dangerous enough to cause bloody diarrhoea [20]. There is a link between water temperature and *E. coli* count. The temperature that is suitable for *E. coli* growth is 20°C to 37°C. A very high or very low temperature is not suitable for the growth of *E. coli*.

Generally, water samples are taken and then the water quality parameters are measured using the suitable methodology and then analysed. Such methods are time-consuming and real-time access to such data is not possible. The Internet of Things (IoT) makes it possible to control any physical device through the internet from any part of the world. There are about 22 water quality parameters [21] and it is not possible to measure all physical and chemical properties of drinking water using the internet of things in real-time and it will cost an enormous amount. But it is possible to measure the prominent water quality parameters using sensors and the internet of things [22]. IoT makes use of water quality sensors, Arduino, NodeMCU, Raspberry Pi 2 or 3, *etc.* for measuring water quality parameters. Sensors are usually analog and need an analog to digital converters (ADC) for transmitting the signals for further analysis. Compared to Arduino or NodeMCU, Raspberry pi has the better computational capability. It is possible to transmit the sensors' values from these low computational devices to database servers. Some analysis algorithms need high computation and memory and for such analysis, data can be accessed directly from these database servers.

A recurrent Neural Network (RNN) is a deep learning network that is commonly used for prediction. Major components of a normal neural network are the input layer, out layer, hidden layer, and an activation function. A deep neural network has hidden units making it more accurate. Long Short Term Memory (LSTM) and Gated Recurrent Unit (GRU) are two types of RNN algorithms. With the help of RNN algorithms, it is possible to predict the changes in water quality parameters.

Smartphones have become an essential part of the day to day life. Smartphones with the Android operating system are sold in large numbers around the world and especially in the Indian market. Global Internet usage is on the rise every day. The main reason for the reduction in the cost of internet data is the competition between Internet service providers, which results in declining Internet data prices . There are new technologies introduced in the smartphone market such as the introduction of 5G networks, the introduction of new mobile processors with high computational capability, *etc.* Recent developments in AngularJS, React, Node.js, and Ionic framework make it possible to create cross-platform native mobile and web applications. This saves the time of coding different applications for android,

IOS, windows, and the web. A single application (Fig. **10**) created using AngularJS or React or Ionic framework runs on any mobile or desktop platform and it also supports responsive design for a better user experience on mobile platforms. Smartphones or tablets can be used by end-users for real-time access to water quality parameters.

METHODS AND MATERIALS

The overall system can be classified into the IoT part and deep learning part (Fig. **1**). Sensors for sensing pH, turbidity, nitrate content, DO and temperature are used in the IoT part. The *E. coli* count cannot be determined directly but temperature acts as an indirect parameter for predicting the favorable conditions for the existence of *E. coli* bacteria. The existence of *E. coli* is much lower at higher and lower temperature levels. The IoT unit (Fig. **2**) is designed for a maximum dimension with 5 feet length, 5 feet width, and 5 feet height overhead tank. The sensors are immersed inside the water level. The unit is especially useful for school overhead tanks and can also be used at other overhead tanks but for larger dimensions, more than one unit of IoT part is needed.

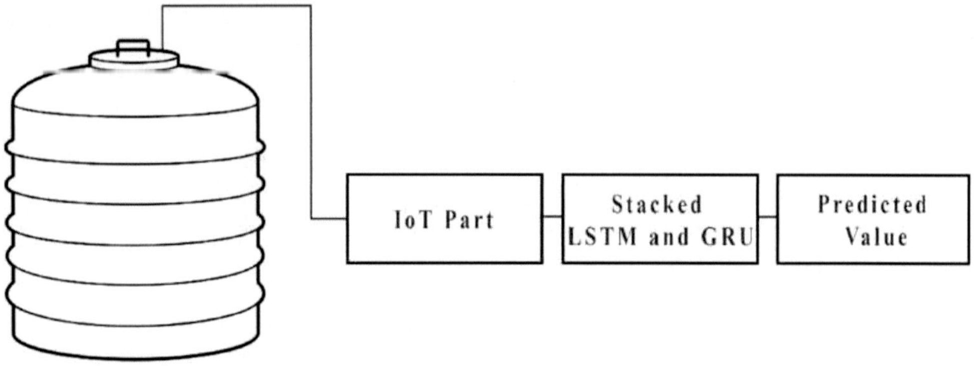

Fig. (1). Schematic diagram of water quality parameters measurement system.

The main components of the IoT unit are pH sensor, nitrate sensor, DO sensor, turbidity sensor, and temperature sensor. The sensors are connected to raspberry pi 4 through an Arduino board. The Arduino board is designed to accept analog signals as input whereas raspberry pi can take only digital signals as input. A suitable interfacing circuit is used for connecting the sensors to the Arduino Uno board. Arduino Uno is a type of microcontroller which is based on 14 digital I/O pins and 6 analog input-output pins. The recommended input voltage for Arduino Uno varies from 7V to 12V. The Arduino Uno is an extremely light-weighted board that weighs around 25 grams [23].

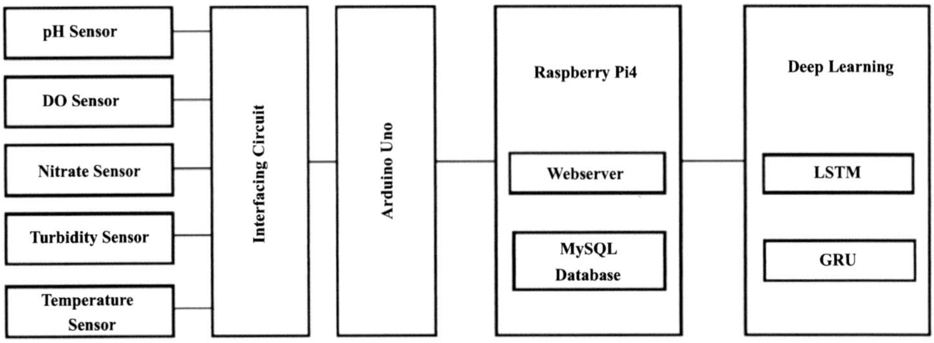

Fig. (2). Internet of things unit.

The Wi-Fi module connected to the Arduino board transmits the sensed data to the raspberry pi board. Raspberry pi has higher computational capability when compared to an Arduino board. The data is transferred between the Arduino and raspberry pi through the Wi-Fi module. Raspberry pi can function as a normal CPU with low computational power. Webserver and MySQL database engine can be installed inside any operating system over the raspberry pi. Sensor data sent from Arduino are stored in the MySQL database.

The IoT units installed at schools or any drinking water overhead tanks are further connected to a cloud server with high computational capability through the internet. Initially, the sensors' data are stored in a local MySQL database, and then the stored data is synchronized with the cloud database at regular intervals. There are other water quality parameters like zinc, a lead that is not sensed by sensors that are manually entered by the authorized authority by direct visits monthly. This ensures that we are considering all water quality parameters for accurate results. The high efficient cloud servers make use of stacked LSTM and GRU for the prediction of water quality parameters.

In recurrent neural networks, gradient finds significant importance. The gradient is referred to as a value that is used to update a neural network's weight. This gradient begins to strain as it propagates through time and its value becomes small and it loses its significance over time, resulting in short-term memory. LSTM and GRU were developed as a solution to the short-term memory problem. Both LSTM and GRU (Fig. **3**) make use of internal gates for regulating and controlling information flow. The gates are important in deciding which information in a sequence is important and needs to be retained and which is not important and needs to be discarded. This process helps to retain relevant information for prediction. In LSTM and GRU, the input data is first transformed into machine-readable vectors after undergoing data pre-processing. While processing these vectors, the previous head's states are transferred consecutively to the next head's state. As the network keeps progressing through states, the hidden values are constantly regulated. The mathematical tanh function helps to regulate the values to always be between -1 to +1.

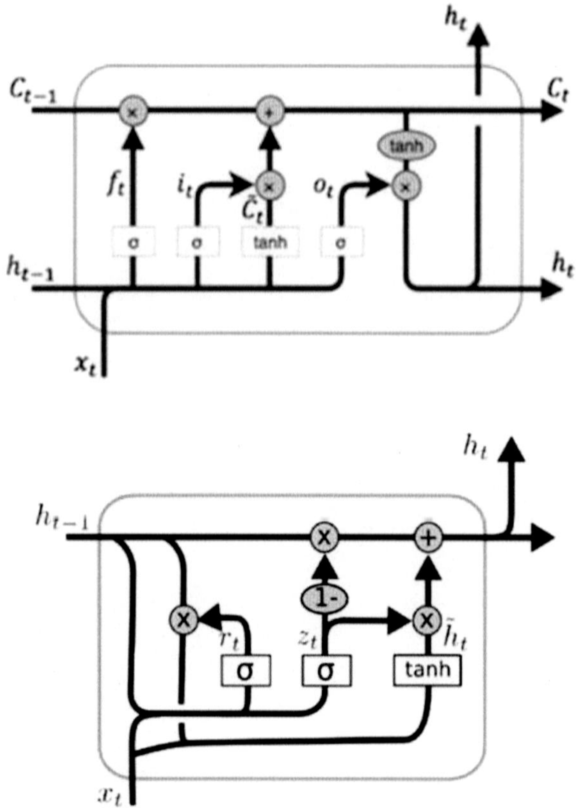

Fig. (3). Structure of LSTM and GRU cells.

The LSTM has the same control flow as a recurrent neural network. The difference is that LSTM makes use of a cell state that helps it to retain or forget the information as data propagates. It also makes use of the sigmoid function which regulates the value between 0 to 1, unlike tanh which varies between -1 and +1. This helps in updating or forgetting data because any multiple of zero is zero. Thus, LSTM makes use of three gates namely input, forget, and an output gate. The data that is to be discarded is sent to the forget gate and data that is to be retained flows through the output gate after undergoing sigmoid and tanh function [24].

$$f_t = \sigma(W_f.(h_{t-1}, x_t) + b_f) \quad (1)$$

$$i_t = \sigma(W_i\ .(h_{t-1}, x_t) + b_i) \quad (2)$$

$$\tilde{C}_t = tanh(\ W_C\ .(h_{t-1}, x_t) +\ b_C\ ) \quad (3)$$

$$C_t = f_t \otimes C_{t-1} +\ i_t \otimes \tilde{C}_t \quad (4)$$

$$o_t = \sigma(\ W_o\ .(\ h_{t-1}, x_t) + b_o\ ) \quad (5)$$

$$h_t =\ o_t \otimes \tanh(C_t) \quad (6)$$

The GRU is a newer generation of RNN. It has two gates namely a reset gate and an update gate [25]. The update gate is similar to that of forget gate in LSTM. It decides the relevant information to retain and irrelevant information to discard. The reset gate is used to decide how information is to be discarded. This makes GRU operate a little faster than LSTM. The best practice is to make use of both LSTM and GRU depending on the use case and make a prediction.

$$z_t = \sigma(\ W_z\ .(h_{t-1}, x_t\ ) \quad (7)$$

$$r_t = \sigma(\ W_r\ .(h_{t-1}, x_t\ ) \quad (8)$$

$$\tilde{h}_t = tanh(W.(r_t \otimes h_{t-1}, x_t)) \quad (9)$$

$$h_t = (1 -\ z_t) \otimes h_{t-1} +\ z_t \otimes \tilde{h}_t \quad (10)$$

Here, the update gate is represented as z_t and the reset gate is represented as r_t.

EXPERIMENTS AND DISCUSSION

We experimented by connecting one IoT unit at Trichy Engineering College and another IoT unit at Surya College of Engineering located at Tiruchirappalli, Tamil Nadu, India. The sensors were initially calibrated using standard solutions for a high degree of accuracy. The Arduino board was connected to a raspberry pi 4 board with 8 GB of RAM, 32 GB of internal storage, and Linux as the operating system. Through the mobile app, manual data entry can be made for lead, zinc, *etc.* through QR code scanning. Experiments have shown that all water quality parameters are within the permissible limits. Since, nitrate is a very important parameter, as it causes fatal diseases such as cancer, we had doped a certain amount of nitrate salt to obtain a greater nitrate value. Dopping of nitrate was carried out in a separate water container so that drinking water was affected. Sensor data was initially stored in the local MySQL database as shown in Table **1**.

Table 1. Sample data of water quality parameters.

S. No.	Site-ID	Time	pH	Nitrate (mg/L)	DO (ppm)	Turb (NTU)	Temp. (ºC)
1	TN001	27-02-2021 12.00.12	6.58	6.3	1.02	0.65	26.1
2	TN002	27-02-2021 12.00.12	6.66	6.35	1.08	0.67	26.46
3	TN001	27-02-2021 13.00.12	6.64	6.42	1.06	0.66	27.3
4	TN002	27-02-2021 13.00.12	6.88	6.45	1.04	0.77	27.9
5	TN001	27-02-2021 14.00.12	6.56	6.62	1.06	0.68	28.1

The stored data was synchronized with a cloud database. Readings were monitored for 60 days and the prediction was made using a stacked LSTM-GRU algorithm with 60 layers of LSTM and 60 layers of GRU and 0.2 dropouts to avoid overfitting. Feature scaling and reshaping were applied to data during data pre-processing. 75% of data was used for training and the remaining 25% of data was used for testing the output. With 50 as batch size, the experiment was done for 600 epochs with adam optimizer and mean squared error loss function.

The actual value and predicted values were plotted in the graph. The graphs show the variation of pH, dissolved oxygen, nitrate, turbidity, and temperature for 60 days along with their predicted values. The variation of pH (Fig. **4**) was between its permissible limit of drinking, which is between 6.5 to 7.5 implies that the pH of the water was good enough to drink. According to the Bureau of Indian Standards (BIS), the pH of the water should be between 6.5 to 8.5 and turbidity (Fig. **5**) should be between 1 to 5 NTU and the following graphs ensure the same.

The dissolved oxygen content of drinking water should be between 0.002 to 2 ppm and too much dissolved oxygen may lead to corrosion of steel pipes [26, 27]. The maximum DO (Fig. **6**) seen was 1.25 ppm. The most important water quality parameter is nitrate concentration and readings of the original water tank were (Fig. **7**) between 6.3 to 6.98 mg/L, which also fell within the 10 mg/L limit.

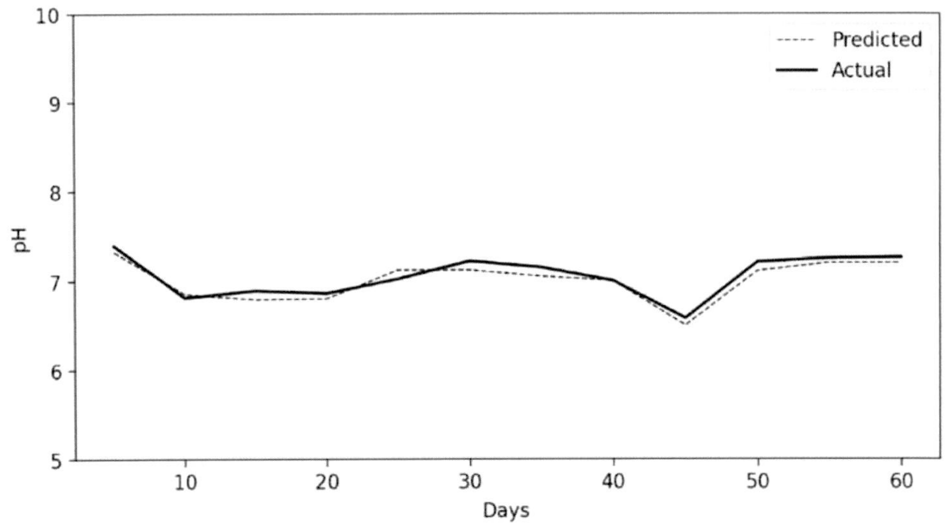

Fig. (4). Variation of pH and its predicted values.

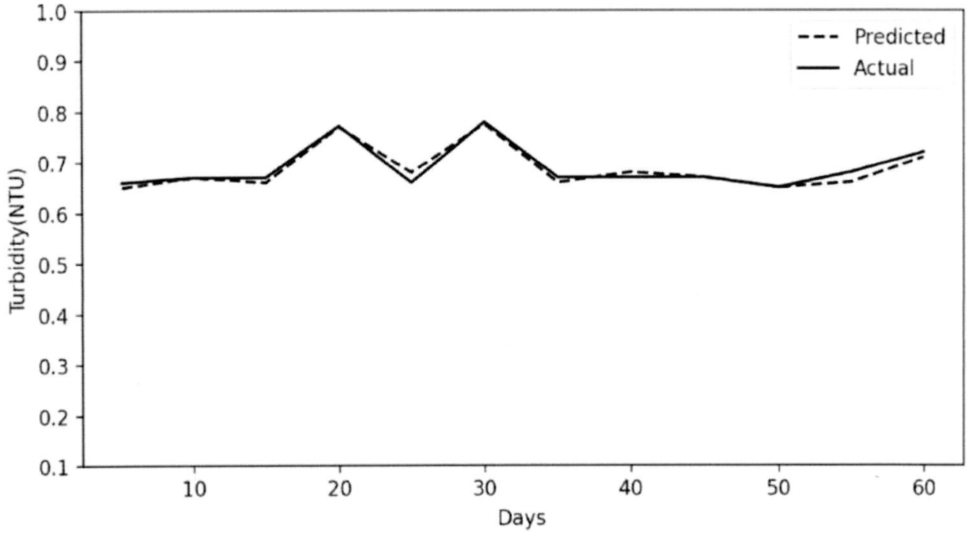

Fig. (5). Variation of turbidity and its predicted values.

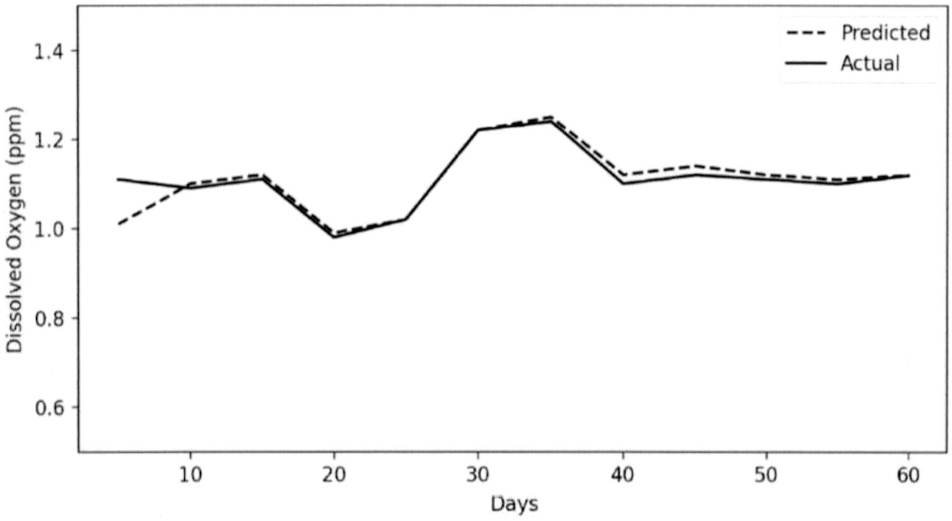

Fig. (6). Variation of dissolved oxygen and its predicted values.

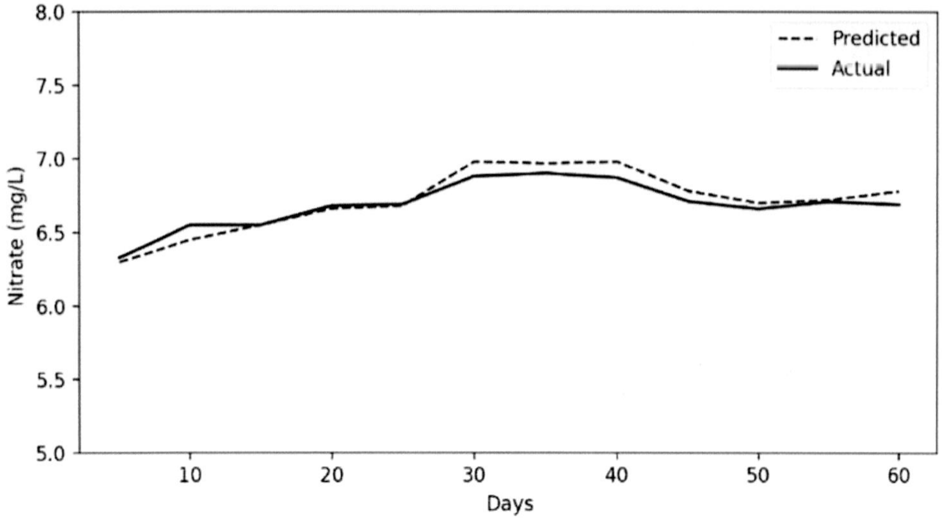

Fig. (7). Variation of nitrate and its predicted values.

The temperature variation (Fig. **8**) was between 25.28°C to 28.55°C. The RMSE (Figs. **9** and **10**) was initially high and RMSE becomes constant after the 300th epoch and the lowest RMSE is 0.07 (Table **2**).

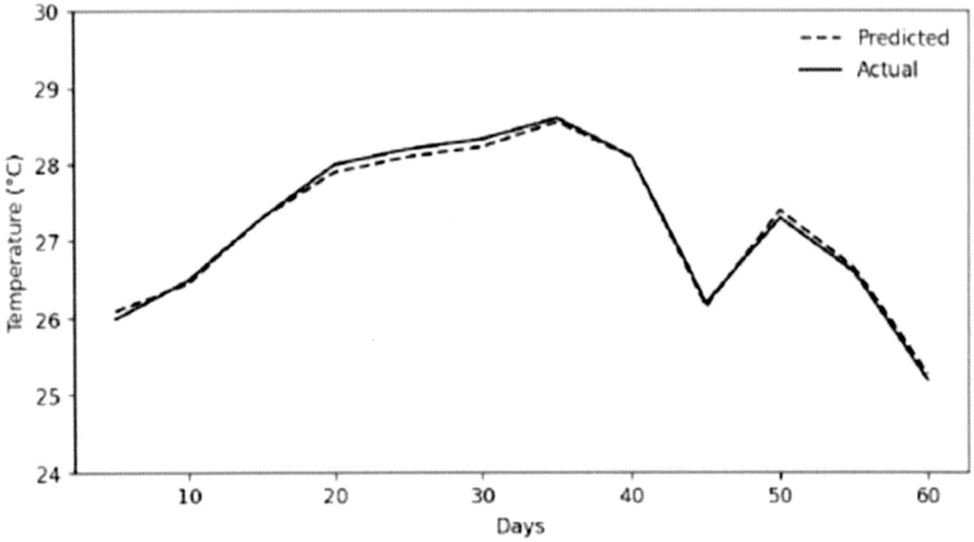

Fig. (8). Variation of temperature and its predicted values.

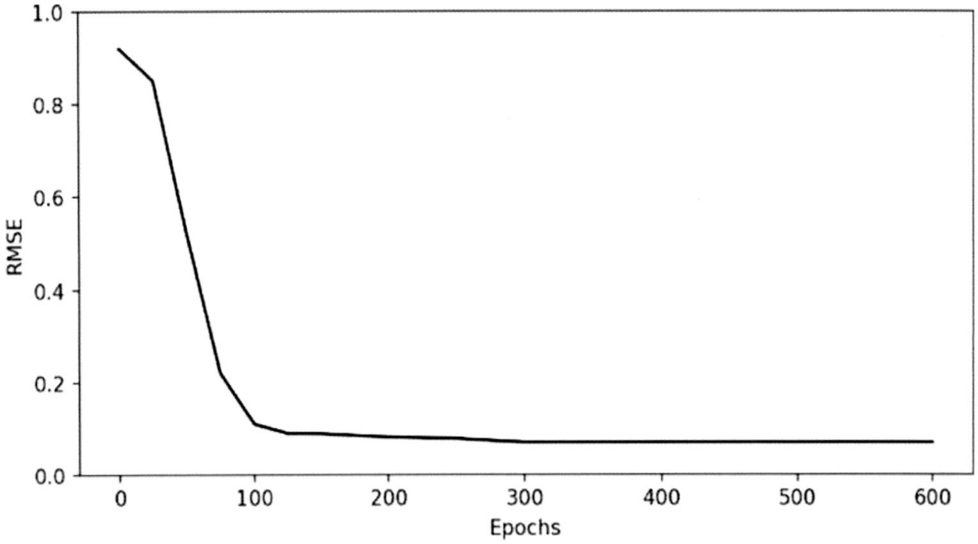

Fig. (9). RMSE *vs.* Epochs.

Table 2. Comparison with existing systems.

Method	Features	RMSE	References
IGRA	DO, Temperature, Precipitation, pH	0.074	[28]
GRU	Dissolved Oxygen	0.411	[29]
Stacked LSTM-GRU	DO, pH, turbidity, temperature, nitrate	0.070	Proposed Method

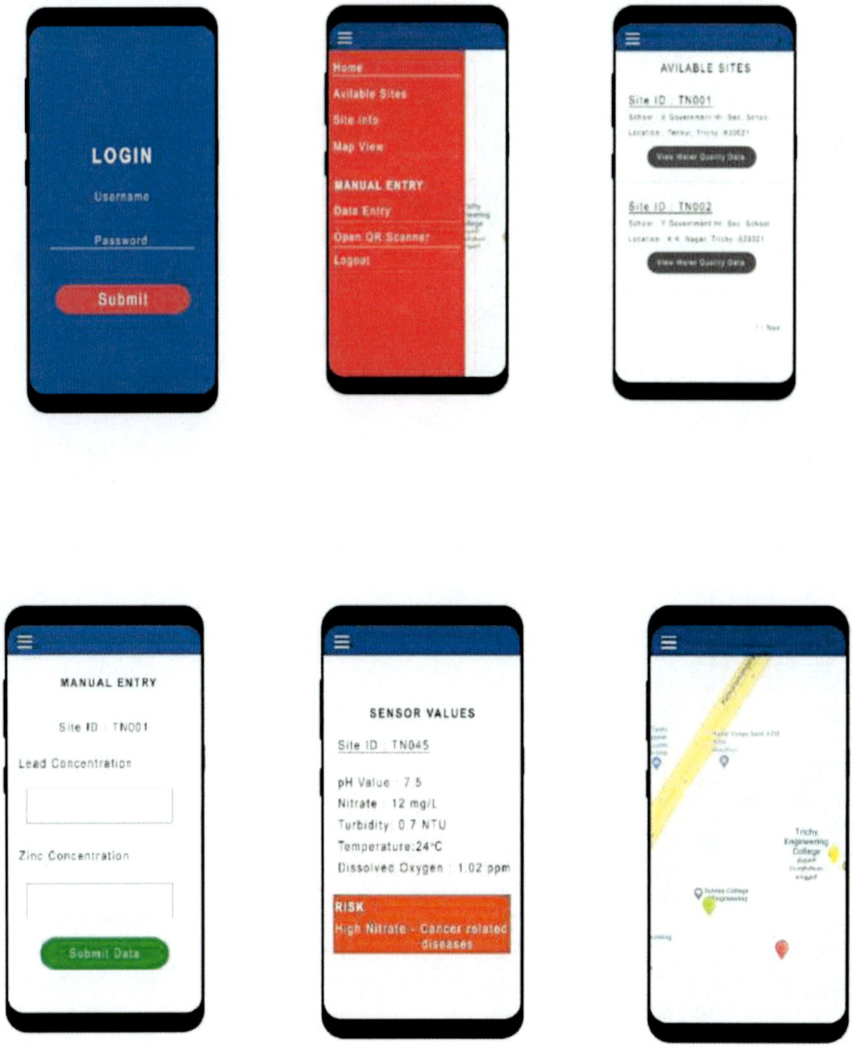

Fig. (10). Mobile interface.

CONCLUSION

Through this, we have implemented a prediction system for water quality parameters. The results show that the predicted values are very close to the actual values. The system can be used by physicians, the public and other authorities to predict water quality parameters for the early detection of water-borne diseases associated with water quality. In near future, other sensors for lead, zinc, *etc.* can be incorporated for more accurate results.

CONSENT FOR PUBLICATION

Not applicable.

CONFLICT OF INTEREST

The author declares no conflict of interest, financial or otherwise.

ACKNOWLEDGEMENT

Declared none.

REFERENCES

[1] N. Adimalla, and H. Qian, "Groundwater quality evaluation using water quality index (WQI) for drinking purposes and human health risk (HHR) assessment in an agricultural region of Nanganur, south India", *Ecotoxicol. Environ. Saf.*, vol. 176, pp. 153-161, 2019. [http://dx.doi.org/10.1016/j.ecoenv.2019.03.066] [PMID: 30927636]

[2] G. Chandrakant, and V. Anantha Rama, "Major Ion Chemistry, Hydro-Geochemical Studies and Mapping of Variability in Ground Water Quality of Sitanadi Basin, Southern Karnataka", *Octa Journal of Environmental Research,* vol. 2, pp. 178-196, 2014.

[3] S.J. Joyce, A. Cook, J. Newnham, M. Brenters, C. Ferguson, and P. Weinstein, "Water disinfection by-products and pre-labor rupture of membranes", *Am. J. Epidemiol.,* vol. 168, no. 5, pp. 514-521, 2008. [http://dx.doi.org/10.1093/aje/kwn188] [PMID: 18635574]

[4] R.K. Ray, T.H. Syed, D. Saha, B.C. Sarkar, and A.K. Patre, "Assessment of village-wise groundwater draft for irrigation: a field-based study in hard-rock aquifers of central India", *Hydrogeol. J.,* vol. 25, no. 8, pp. 2513-2525, 2017. [http://dx.doi.org/10.1007/s10040-017-1625-x]

[5] J.G. Brody, A. Aschengrau, W. McKelvey, C.H. Swartz, T. Kennedy, and R.A. Rudel, "Breast cancer risk and drinking water contaminated by wastewater: a case control study", *Environ. Health,* vol. 5, no. 1, p. 28, 2006. [http://dx.doi.org/10.1186/1476-069X-5-28] [PMID: 17026759]

[6] M. Inoue-Choi, R.R. Jones, K.E. Anderson, K.P. Cantor, J.R. Cerhan, S. Krasner, K. Robien, P.J. Weyer, and M.H. Ward, "Nitrate and nitrite ingestion and risk of ovarian cancer among postmenopausal women in Iowa", *Int. J. Cancer,* vol. 137, no. 1, pp. 173-182, 2015. [http://dx.doi.org/10.1002/ijc.29365] [PMID: 25430487]

[7] J.A. McElroy, A. Trentham-Dietz, R.E. Gangnon, J.M. Hampton, A.J. Bersch, M.S. Kanarek, and P.A. Newcomb, "Nitrogen-nitrate exposure from drinking water and colorectal cancer risk for rural women in Wisconsin, USA", *J. Water Health,* vol. 6, no. 3, pp. 399-409, 2008. [http://dx.doi.org/10.2166/wh.2008.048] [PMID: 19108561]

[8] B.A. Mueller, S. Searles Nielsen, S. Preston-Martin, E.A. Holly, S. Cordier, G. Filippini, R. Peris-Bonet, and N.W. Choi, "Household water source and the risk of childhood brain tumours: results of the SEARCH International Brain Tumor Study", *Int. J. Epidemiol.,* vol. 33, no. 6, pp. 1209-1216, 2004. [http://dx.doi.org/10.1093/ije/dyh215] [PMID: 15567873]

[9] A.J.L. Quist, M. Inoue-Choi, P.J. Weyer, K.E. Anderson, K.P. Cantor, S. Krasner, L.E.B. Freeman, M.H. Ward, and R.R. Jones, "Ingested nitrate and nitrite, disinfection by-products, and pancreatic cancer risk in postmenopausal women", *Int. J. Cancer,* vol. 142, no. 2, pp. 251-261, 2018. [http://dx.doi.org/10.1002/ijc.31055] [PMID: 28921575]

[10] M.H. Ward, E.F. Heineman, R.S. Markin, and D.D. Weisenburger, "Adenocarcinoma of the stomach and esophagus and drinking water and dietary sources of nitrate and nitrite", *Int. J. Occup. Environ. Health,* vol. 14, no. 3, pp. 193-197, 2008. [http://dx.doi.org/10.1179/oeh.2008.14.3.193] [PMID: 18686719]

[11] M.H. Ward, J.A. Rusiecki, C.F. Lynch, and K.P. Cantor, "Nitrate in public water supplies and the risk of renal cell carcinoma", *Cancer Causes Control,* vol. 18, no. 10, pp. 1141-1151, 2007. [http://dx.doi.org/10.1007/s10552-007-9053-1] [PMID: 17717631]

[12] M.P. Zeegers, R.F.M. Selen, J.C.S. Kleinjans, R.A. Goldbohm, and P.A. van den Brandt, "Nitrate intake does not influence bladder cancer risk: the Netherlands cohort study", *Environ. Health Perspect.,* vol. 114, no. 10, pp. 1527-1531, 2006. [http://dx.doi.org/10.1289/ehp.9098] [PMID: 17035137]

[13] M. Albouy-Llaty, F. Limousi, C. Carles, A. Dupuis, S. Rabouan, and V. Migeot, "Association between Exposure to Endocrine Disruptors in Drinking Water and Preterm Birth, Taking Neighborhood Deprivation into Account: A Historic Cohort Study", *Int. J. Environ. Res. Public Health,* vol. 13, no. 8, p. 796, 2016. [http://dx.doi.org/10.3390/ijerph13080796] [PMID: 27517943]

[14] S.J. Joyce, A. Cook, J. Newnham, M. Brenters, C. Ferguson, and P. Weinstein, "Water disinfection by-products and pre-labor rupture of membranes", *Am. J. Epidemiol.,* vol. 168, no. 5, pp. 514-521, 2008. [http://dx.doi.org/10.1093/aje/kwn188] [PMID: 18635574]

[15] K.D. Mattix, P.D. Winchester, and L.R.T. Scherer, "Incidence of abdominal wall defects is related to surface water atrazine and nitrate levels", *J. Pediatr. Surg.,* vol. 42, no. 6, pp. 947-949, 2007. [http://dx.doi.org/10.1016/j.jpedsurg.2007.01.027] [PMID: 17560200]

[16] S.A. Waller, K. Paul, S.E. Peterson, and J.E. Hitti, "Agricultural-related chemical exposures, season of conception, and risk of gastroschisis in Washington State", *Obstet. Gynecol. Surv.,* vol. 202, no. 3, pp. 241.e1-241.e6, 2010. [PMID: 20207240]

[17] A.G. Mann, C.C. Tam, C.D. Higgins, and L.C. Rodrigues, "The association between drinking water turbidity and gastrointestinal illness: a systematic review", *BMC Public Health,* vol. 7, no. 1, p. 256, 2007. [http://dx.doi.org/10.1186/1471-2458-7-256] [PMID: 17888154]

[18] F. Greenway, *Faculty Opinions Recommendation of Potential Benefits of PH 8.8 Alkaline Drinking Water as an Adjunct in the Treatment of Reflux Disease.* Faculty Opinions – Post-Publication Peer Review of the Biomedical Literature, 2013. [http://dx.doi.org/10.3410/f.718021982.793479080]

[19] A. Jan, M. Azam, K. Siddiqui, A. Ali, I. Choi, and Q. Haq, "Heavy Metals and Human Health: Mechanistic Insight into Toxicity and Counter Defense System of Antioxidants", *Int. J. Mol. Sci.,* vol. 16, no. 12, pp. 29592-29630, 2015. [http://dx.doi.org/10.3390/ijms161226183] [PMID: 26690422]

[20] S.T. Odonkor, and T. Mahami, "Escherichia coli as a Tool for Disease Risk Assessment of Drinking Water Sources", *Int. J. Microbiol.,* vol. 2020, pp. 1-7, 2020. [http://dx.doi.org/10.1155/2020/2534130] [PMID: 32612658]

[21] A.K. Chaurasia, H.K. Pandey, S.K. Tiwari, R. Prakash, P. Pandey, and A. Ram, "Groundwater Quality assessment using Water Quality Index (WQI) in parts of Varanasi District, Uttar Pradesh, India", *J. Geol. Soc. India,* vol. 92, no. 1, pp. 76-82, 2018. [http://dx.doi.org/10.1007/s12594-018-0955-1]

[22] S. Geetha, and S. Gouthami, "Internet of Things Enabled Real Time Water Quality Monitoring System", *Smart Water,* vol. 2, no. 1, 2016. [http://dx.doi.org/10.1186/s40713-017-0005-y]

[23] A.A. Galadima, "Arduino as a Learning Tool", *11th International Conference on Electronics, Computer and Computation (ICECCO)* 2014.

[24] S. Hochreiter, and J. Schmidhuber, "Long short-term memory", *Neural Comput.,* vol. 9, no. 8, pp. 1735-1780, 1997.
[http://dx.doi.org/10.1162/neco.1997.9.8.1735] [PMID: 9377276]

[25] K. Cho, B. van Merrienboer, C. Gulcehre, D. Bahdanau, F. Bougares, H. Schwenk, and Y. Bengio, "Learning Phrase Representations Using RNN Encoder-Decoder for Statistical Machine Translation", *Proceedings of the 2014 Conference on Empirical Methods in Natural Language Processing (EMNLP)* 2014.
[http://dx.doi.org/10.3115/v1/D14-1179]

[26] K.V. Rybalka, L.A. Beketaeva, and A.D. Davydov, "Effect of Dissolved Oxygen on the Corrosion Rate of Stainless Steel in a Sodium Chloride Solution", *Russ. J. Electrochem.,* vol. 54, no. 12, pp. 1284-1287, 2018.
[http://dx.doi.org/10.1134/S1023193518130384]

[27] G. Dirisu Chimezie, M.O. Mafiana, G.B. Dirisu, and R. Amodu, "Level of PH in Drinking Water of an Oil and Gas Producing Community and Perceived Biological and Health Implications", *European Journal of Basic and Applied Sciences,* vol. 3, no. 3, pp. 2059-3058, 2016.

[28] J. Zhou, Y. Wang, F. Xiao, Y. Wang, and L. Sun, "Water Quality Prediction Method Based on IGRA and LSTM", *Water,* vol. 10, no. 9, p. 1148, 2018.
[http://dx.doi.org/10.3390/w10091148]

[29] W. Li, H. Wu, N. Zhu, Y. Jiang, J. Tan, and Y. Guo, "Prediction of dissolved oxygen in a fishery pond based on gated recurrent unit (GRU)", *Inf. Process. Agric.,* vol. 8, no. 1, pp. 185-193, 2021.
[http://dx.doi.org/10.1016/j.inpa.2020.02.002]

CHAPTER 9

IoT-Enabled Crowd Monitoring and Control to Avoid Covid Disease Spread Using Crowdnet and YOLO

Sujatha Rajkumar[1], **Sameer Ahamed R.**[1], **Srinija Ramichetty**[1,*] and **Eshita Suri**[1]

[1] *Vellore Institute of Technology, Vellore, Tamil Nadu, India*

Abstract: COVID-19 is an infectious disease that has spread globally, and the best way to slow down transmission is to maintain a safe distance. Due to the COVID-19 spread, social distancing has become very vital. Furthermore, the formation of groups and crowds cannot be left unseen. Even when the necessary regulations have been implemented by governments worldwide, people tend not to follow the rules. We wanted to make it possible for authorities in areas like schools, universities, industries, hospitals, restaurants, *etc.*, to monitor people breaking social distancing rules and take appropriate measures to control the virus from spreading. To monitor and control the crowd, society requires a system that does not put other people's lives at risk. Therefore, it is critical that we stop it from spreading further. Initially, the government imposed a lockdown to control the spread of the virus. Due to the lockdowns, the economy had experienced some negative effects. Due to the economic slowdown, people were allowed to go out and carry on with their regular tasks, leading to crowding in many places, intentionally or unintentionally. The research work aims to make a crowd detection and alert system in public places like hospitals, schools, universities, and other public gathering events. The proposed idea has two modules; a deep CNN CrowdNet people counting algorithm to detect the distance between humans in highly dense crowds and an IoT platform for sending information to the authorities whenever there is a violation. Image processing is carried out in two parts: extraction of frames from real-time videos using YOLO CV, and the second is processing the frame to detect the number of people in the crowd.

The crowd counting algorithm, along with the vaccination, will enforce safety rules in people-gathering places and minimize health risks and spread. The image processing YOLO model mainly targets people not following social distancing norms and standing very close by. The data for the violations are sent online to the IoT platform, where the value is compared to a threshold. The platform aids in sending alerts to the concerned authorities in case of significant violations. Warnings are sent through e-mail or personal messages to the concerned authorities and the location.

* **Corresponding author Srinija Ramichetty:** Vellore Institute of Technology, Vellore, Tamil Nadu, India; Tel: +9186100 45822; E-mail: srinija.ramichetty2018@vitstudent.ac.in

Sivakumar R., Dimiter Velev, Basim Alhadidi, S. Vidhya, Sheeja V. Francis and B. Prabadevi (Eds.)

This model prevents the presence of an official to check whom all are violating the rules. There is no need for human intervention and risking their lives; direct messages can be sent through the IoT platform to authorities if there is a crowd formation. Data analytics can help find out the peak hours of crowding and help control the crowd much more efficiently. CrowdNet, a deep CNN algorithm, will estimate the number of humans in a given frame to classify the locations where most people communicate and check whether the safe distance is not reached and the number of times it is not reached. Our system sends the number of people available in the frame at that moment and whether they are maintaining social distancing or not. The Deep CNN algorithm will filter the objects by capturing high-level semantics required to count only the humans and calculate the distance between the humans alone. The base neural network is Alexnet to estimate whether it is safe or not and then send it to the respective authority. This proposed idea using CrowdNet CNN and IoT combination will help find out peak hours of crowding and help control the spread of the disease during social distance violations without human intervention. Thus, social distancing in public places is automated using the real-time deep learning-based framework *via* object detection, tracking, and controlled disease.

Keywords: COCO, Convolutional Neural Networks (CNN), CrowdNet, Social Distancing, Ubidots, YOLO.

INTRODUCTION

The Coronavirus pandemic hit the world in the first week of March last year. It was long before 2020 when it began and spread. The initial spread can be attributed to lower test cases and virtually no social distancing. It is reported by Medical News Today that close distance means staying close to 6 feet from the nearest person. By the first week of March, it had spread to 90 countries. By mid-march, WHO declared it a global pandemic, and more than 115 countries declared it a national emergency state. While most healthcare organizations and medical experts were trying to develop an effective method to prevent the exponential growth of covid cases, the cases kept growing, and the death rates skyrocketed. Responding to this, the countries decided on lockdown and curfews to implement social distancing.

To maintain and improve our economy, working under social distancing was the only solution. A considerable disadvantage of lockdown is that it badly affects the economy, and livelihood of the people. In an article, the world economic forum stated that close to 114 million people lost their jobs due to COVID-19 making it the worst ever. For those who did not lose their jobs, salaries were cut. Business sectors like tourism and transport were enormously affected. Many cab drivers were not earning their payday. This raised anxiety and tension for the people to search for jobs and provide for their families again. Presently we can observe that markets and opportunities have started to open. Now, it will be an incentive for corporations, employers, and employees to collectively make an effort to maximize social distancing, minimizing social contact with others. This can only be tackled and succeeded collectively. Ensuring social distancing will decrease the cases drastically, and jobs and livelihood can turn back to normal. This research project aims to scrutinize different algorithms and find an effective social distancing measure among the masses.

Background of the Research Work

The current research utilizes Raspberry Pi 4 with 4 GB RAM for running the code, following rationale such as ARM Cortex A-72 as the processor- the A series of ARM processors are best to run Machine learning. Specifically, A-72 is intensively designed and used for running computer vision algorithms. It also has a high computed density and advanced branch predictor, making Raspberry Pi the best choice for our use case. The input is taken as a video for Raspberry Pi using raspberry-pi camera v1. The camera is capable of producing 5 Megapixel OmniVision resolution pictures and videos. The camera also supports 1080 pixel resolution with 30 frames per second, 720-pixel resolution with 60 frames per second, and 640* 480-pixel resolution for 60/90 recording. Currently, we are using 1080 pixel resolution with 30 frames per second for our video throughput. The Raspberry Pi 4 has a Broadcom BCM2711 SoC, which provides GPIO access and helps manage the devices like the camera. The current Raspberry Pi camera communicates on the CSI bus with the BCM2711 processor.

For processing the captured images, deep learning object detection techniques are used. Nowadays, many methods like detection-based, feature-regression-based, cluster-based, and neural network-based are available for crowd counting and object detection. A convolutional neural network (CNN) which consists of many hidden layers, is used for object detection. This is done by drawing bounding boxes around the object of interest. Feedforward neural networks or MLPs were among the first methods of object detection. However, due to certain limitations, it used many regions to detect and classify objects, which required considerable computational time, making it unsuitable for real-time object detection. To avoid this, Region-based convolutional neural networks, which extract about 2000 region proposals from an image, are favoured. Regional-based Convolutional Neural Network (RCNN) identifies these specific regions based on four parameters- colours, textures, varying scales, and enclosure. These parameters form a specific pattern recognized by the neural network and taken up as regions. Once the regions are extracted, they are resized and reshaped to match the input size of the CNN model. After that, this high-capacity CNN extracts a fixed-length feature vector from each region and forwards it to a set of class-specific, linear-specific vector machines (SVMs). The feature extractor is AlexNet since it can support an extensive model and utilizes very little time for training.

Further, one binary SVM for each class is trained to classify the required object and the background. Our paper uses the You only look once (YOLO) model because of its well-performing architecture for object detection and high fps in real-time usage. It is a clever algorithm with high accuracy, and this accuracy is achieved because it uses a single forward propagation pass to make the predictions. This algorithm is based on classification and is implemented in two stages. Firstly, an ROI (region of interest) is defined, and these selected regions are then classified.

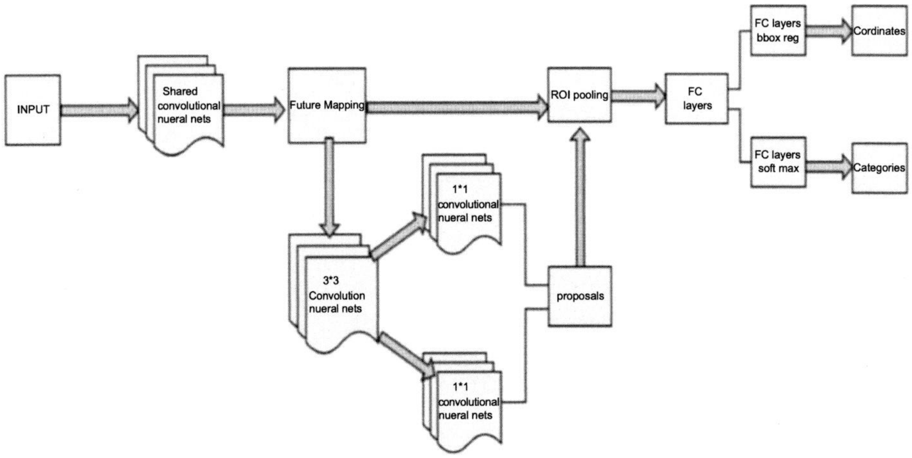

Fig. (1). YOLO model.

From Fig. (**1**), we can infer that YOLO divides the entire image into an equal number of grids, and different parameters like confidence and weights are considered to detect the object required in our use case. For example, if we want to detect the centre of the object we are looking for, that particular grid's confidence should be around or equal to 1. Upon the confidence, we can move on the grids considering x, and y as the object's coordinates or the centre of the object to be detected. Later if there are more objects in a particular frame, all of them are considered into different classes, and a softmax function is applied to extract the particular class, and finally, we construct our neural network to make the required predictions. Once the objects are successfully sorted into classes, bounding boxes specifying their location are included. Since the paper talks about a comparative study, another deep CNN algorithm called CrowdNet is studied simultaneously.

CrowdNet is a convolutional neural network that detects and estimates crowd density from a given dataset or live feed. CrowdNet is a flexible tool that takes into account the perspective of the camera in the environment. Given a hypothetical situation, a person who stands near the camera can be detected easily as his head with his body is present. The person is visible when he is near. As the distance between the camera and the person increases, we then can only rely on a few pixels gathering the data to detect the person. CrowdNet uses a deep and shallow network depending upon the above situation. The scenario given uses a shallow network to detect a person who is relatively far away from the camera and a deep network to detect a person relatively near. This provides CrowdNet with its hybrid nature and flexibility. The architectural design deep network uses is closely comparable to the VGG-16 network. The purpose of VGG-16 is to classify everyday objects like chairs, bicycles, sofas, and cars. The VGG-16 architecture has five max-pool layers. Each of the max-pool layers in the VGG-16 architecture has two strides. There is only 1/32th spatial resolution when an input image is inserted.

On the other hand, the shallow network is used to detect tiny heads in a massive crowd. The complexity of detecting only the head is lower when compared to deep networks. This is because the pixel information that is taken by the shallow network is minimally comparatively. The shallow layer only uses three convolutional layers for its detection. The size of each kernel in each of these layers is 5x5, which uses twenty-four filters. To improve the accuracy, an average of all the pooling layers is taken.

Literature Survey

Dongfang *et al.* [1] developed a non-intrusive augmentative AI-based surveillance system. The desired outcomes include a novel vision-based real-time social distancing and crowd density detection. The statistical approach incorporated uses a monocular camera to detect individuals in a region of interest (ROI), and the real-time data collected is used to calculate the interpersonal distances between people. A deep CNN model YOLO is used to detect the pedestrians in the image domain, and then by using the mapping functions, the image coordinates are mapped into real-world coordinates. These coordinates are then used in the Euclidean distance formula. Finally, to find the critical social density, a simple linear regression is performed on the collected data.

Pertiwang *et al.* [2] proposed a system where the comparison of identifying and processing the human image is primarily based on the algorithms "YOLOLITE" and "YOLOV3". Computer vision (CV) is a branch of computer science that explores how algorithms can be taught to perceive and interpret photo data in the same way we do. OpenCV is just one of many accessible, open-source CV frameworks that have been proposed. The whole article presents and analyses the efficiency of the YOLO-LITE as well as YOLOV3 algorithms. Both algorithms have been applied in many real-time tests, all of which were carried out in the same test environment. According to Alex *et al.*, the Raspberry Pi camera operated at Fifteen frames per second with YOLO-LITE and One frame per second with YOLOV3 [3]. The convolutional neural network (CNN) that was trained to identify 1.2 million high-resolution photos among thousand separate categories is discussed. This has been done as a part of the ImageNet LSVRC-2010 competition. The network has 5 convolutional layers and 3 completely connected layers in its framework. The following are innovative architectural features: The network comprises eight layers, each of which includes certain weights. The first five are convolution layers, while the remaining three are related. While the last completely connected layers are fed as an input to a thousand-way softmax feature, approximately 1000 classifiers are generated. Only the second, fourth, and fifth convolution layer is related to the kernel maps of the previous layer since they are all on the same Graphical Processing Unit. A batch size of 128 samples was used. These models are trained to employ stochastic gradient descent, momentum and weight decay. Furthermore, the model's ability to learn is aided by this tiny amount of weight loss. In other words, weight decay is not just a regularizer but also decreases the model's classification error.

Mayur *et al.* [4] analyses in-depth calculating density calculation, finding a region of motion, and crowd detection. It uses a Deep Convolutional Neural Network process that considers different approaches like Detection-based, Regression-based, and Density-based. This paper looks at an efficient method that takes end-to-end training, uses the whole image, and performs inference. Since our project's primary aim is to detect a crowd indoors, we do not expect to have a group in a mass gathering. Therefore, it is understood and extracted the crux of their approach to crowd detection and simplified it to our indoor application.

Kumar *et al.* [5] discusses a novel method to track humans in a harsh environment. They used pre-recorded footage (not real-time data) to detect and track a human frame by frame. They can do this because of a. The paper discusses two ways to trace a human, namely Detection and Tracking. The algorithm proposed uses a variety of detection and tracking. Their model uses 3 Convolutional Neural Networks (which are based on Deep learning) to improve the overall effectiveness of their model. They have expanded and gone out to test their model of other types of objects such as (football, woman, boy, and basketball). Although this model is robust, it costs considerable processing power to make this Algorithm run. Therefore, this can only run on specialized and power systems. We aim to present an idea that can work on low-power devices, such as a Raspberry Pi. Another improvement possible with the paper is to take real-time data and train the algorithm [6].

Giovanna *et al.* [7] poses an innovative use of crowd detection. Although this paper has a specific application to land drones in a safe spot, it nevertheless uses crowd detection techniques to achieve that purpose. Using a drone comes with many constraints. To mention a few, drones will have a limited processing capability, and the proposed algorithm should be of small processing capability. The advantage of this paper compared to other papers in this field is that there is a constraint on mobility and efficiency in the use of power when designing an algorithm for crowd detection. This paper discusses a two-loss model, lightweight FCN architecture. The model contains two different tasks, namely classification and regression. The regression task is aided and applied after the classification task, which is used to segregate between densely/loosely packed scenes aimed at drastically pinpointing the agglomeration tendency of the crowd present there. The paper can be enhanced by using a real data set to train the system. Instead, the system has only been trained by sample datasets. Also, the paper can work on improving accuracy as the components and processing limits in a drone are seriously low.

Mamoona *et al.* [8] presented a novel in this algorithm, took account of an image, and then divided it into smaller rectangular sub-sections. They used a Convolutional Neural Network head detector. After each of the rectangular subsection images has been obtained, the algorithm then decides whether there is a crowd/No crowd in each of the subsection images using the SURF binary feature SVM classifier. The algorithm mainly focuses on the head directions as the head is the most prominently visible body part in a sea of people. For the subsection images where no images have been detected, they used neighbouring pixels to find a weighted average of that model. This model can be improved if we use a better algorithm like YOLO. Also, the information perspective of the image taken is not accounted for. We can create a formula to feed in the perspective of the camera so that processing can be far more efficient. Lastly, the system is checked against three datasets only. We can use far more data sets to train and make sure that the system is as accurate as possible [9].

Hamid *et al.* [10] discusses the usage of MIST computing instead of cloud computing. MIST computing is mainly based on Fog computing, but the computational servers are more scattered than the Fog computing servers. MIST computing is primarily used in Image processing applications because the data is bigger, and implementing applications on the data leads to increased latency in the operation of the Image processing model. MIST computing can be used in our project by uploading the Image processing algorithm on the microcontroller board and connecting it to the local CCTV camera. The microcontroller board will also be able to communicate the alerts to the local authorities using its internet connectivity.

Dan *et al.* [11] built a device that uses a single camera to count people in masses. The normalization approach is used to deal with viewpoints and various camera orientations. As a result, the recommended system is successfully trained to be an independent viewpoint system and introduced to a new site with minimal setup. It indicates that every other frame has been subjected to the technique of context subtraction and edge detection, as well as the extraction of edge orientation. A homograph is calculated between the surface plane and object plane coordinates to measure the area of interest. A distribution map that calculates person size and then a global scale that calculates camera alignment are computed and used for feature normalization. The supervised learning data can then be used to find and evaluate the correlation between function histograms and the number of people throughout the crowds. The linear fitting and neural network approaches are used in this article. One significant change integrated into our article is that, since we will not be counting pedestrians, once the training is completed, we will be able to launch the framework for online mass counting immediately.

Afnan *et al.* [12] ensemble a framework based on free software and easily accessible sensors. This installation is perfect for stores and institutions because it includes a non-contact thermal temperature sensor (MLX90614) that analyses the thermal temperature of a human body that enters the room, the very following functionality is queueing up the individuals using a VL531x time of flight (ToF) sensor in combination with WS2812B addressable LEDs. Ultimately, a Raspberry Pi broad-angle camera module is then used to detect breaches. The tunable LEDs serve as the camera's reference markers, and the device sends out a warning if anyone crosses them. Presently, this device can only be used to search for infringement within the designated areas.

Nurul *et al.* [13], solely focuses on YOLOv3 to detect humans. YOLO means that You Only Look Once. This is a relatively new technique that cuts the algorithm into different regions. Then the probability of each of the regions is calculated. The authors also speak about maximizing the utilization of the GPU, as it is challenging to do so. The mAP acquired from their tests is equal to 78.3%. This algorithm is generally similar to other CNN algorithms. Using an improved processor, we could improve the accuracy and efficiency of the proposed model. This is the most efficient processing algorithm we have seen in a literature review, as this is an extended and efficient version of the previous YOLOv3 algorithm [14, 15].

According to Marco *et al.* [16], a surveillance system that was explicitly designed to track static swarmed scenes is depicted. The study focused on static communities formed by clumps of people who gathered and stayed in the same place for an extended period. The definition of fixed groups is achieved with the aid of a One-Class Support Vector Machine. Surface highlights that were removed at the fixing stage are chipped away. Spatial regions containing groups could be easily identified and segregated using movement data, avoiding the creation of clamour and false alarms resulting from people's continuous movement. It is possible to obtain, from one given preparing the package, an adequately summarised model of categories that can be implemented for each of the situations sharing a comparative perspective using one category grouping and internal surface descriptors. Because the aim was to use different approaches and methods for social events from streams or individuals walking down the street, both surface and activity data were abused. The use of One-Class SVM allowed the system to become more familiar only with necessary limits. As a result, it is very easy to summarise the configurations with similar review points [17, 18].

According to Rachel *et al.* [19], YOLO-LITE is used in this article. The whole model is used to detect objects in an image and has the added benefit of being able to operate on mobile devices without a Graphics Card, such as a laptop or a smartphone (GPU). The PASCAL VOC database was used to construct the model at first, and then the COCO database was introduced later, yielding mAPs of 33.81 per cent and 12.26 per cent, respectively. YOLO-LITE also has an advantage over the broader YOLO architecture in that it features some of the fastest object detection algorithms. On non-GPU processors, they are hardly real-time (2.4 FPS), despite being much faster than the more significant YOLO architecture. YOLO-LITE also makes a unique contribution to image recognition by demonstrating that shallow networks do have a great deal of potential for compact real-time image recognition networks and that operating at 21 frames per second on a non-GPU device is very impressive for such a small system.

Geethapriya *et al.* [20] discusses the YOLO algorithm for detecting objects using a single neural network. This algorithm is organized. It outflanks various techniques once summing up from natural pictures to various domains. The algorithm is easy to construct and can be prepared straightforwardly on a total image. Region proposal systems limit the classifier to a specific area. YOLO gets to the whole picture in anticipating limits. Furthermore, it predicts fewer false positives in background areas. Compared to another classifier algorithm, this algorithm is a substantially more productive and quickest algorithm to use progressively.

According to Tanvir *et al.* [21], in object detection, recently, success has been accomplished at a big scale, yet at the same time, it is quite a challenging task to detect and identify objects accurately and at a fast speed. This paper proposes a modified YOLOv1-based neural network for object detection. The new neural network model has been improved in the following ways. Firstly, the loss function of the YOLOv1 network is modified, and the improved model replaces the margin style with the proportion style. This modified version of the loss function is more flexible and more reasonable in optimizing the network error. Secondly, a spatial pyramid pooling layer is added; thirdly, an inception model with a convolution kernel of 1 * 1 is added, which helps in reducing the total number of weight parameters present in the layers. Extensive experiments on Pascal VOC datasets 2007/ 2012 showed that the proposed method achieved better performance.

YOLO Model for Crowd Detection

YOLO is a classification-based algorithm that is used for object detection. It applies a single convolutional neural network to the entire image, which divides the image into regions. These grids or regions are created to predict the bounding boxes. The bounding boxes are a set of rectangular boxes that enclose the object that is to be detected. In our article, these bounding boxes enclose the humans, and then by applying the formula of euclidean distance between these boxes, the distance between the individuals is calculated. COCO is a labelled dataset that was created by Microsoft in 2014. This dataset is used widely for tasks like captioning, object detection, stuff image segmentation, *etc.* When used for object detection, the dataset has annotations for bounding boxes and pre-labelled segmentation masks for about 80 categories. These categories are the different objects that we use in everyday life, and we are using this dataset in our project to detect humans. UBIDOTS is the IoT platform that is used to show the real-time data taken by the YOLO model. The data collected or the number of people detected is shown as a dashboard. Another feature offered by this platform is that it lets us analyze previously collected data. It is also used to send an alert in the form of a message and a mail to the concerned authorities when the crowd density crosses the previously set threshold value. The TensorFlow is an open-source developed for easy implementation of machine learning models with its inbuilt libraries. The TensorFlow follows three phases in its architecture data preprocessing, constructing the model, and training the model as required by the test data set. The TensorFlow, in our case, takes in considerable input and helps train our CNN model. OpenCV is an open-source library that will be used to capture the video and perform the image processing techniques. It will convert the captured video into a set of images on which we can apply the object detection model. We are running YOLO on Raspberry Pi. Raspberry Pi is a sophisticated mini board that can perform the functionalities of a computer, for example, running an operating system like Linux. The provision of GPIO pins on the board helps us interface different peripherals like sensors, cameras, other boards, *etc.* The board also provides 2 types of USB interfaces and a memory card slot to store the sensor data. In the current project, Raspberry Pi is used to run the code related to the YOLO algorithm and CrowdNet algorithm based on the input provided by the Raspberry Pi camera. The small form factor and low power requirements make this board perfect for running the algorithms mentioned above. Raspberry Pi Camera V1 module is a custom-made module for Raspberry Pi. This allows the camera to interact with the Raspberry Pi board firmware easily. The camera module gets interfaced with the board through a CSI interface. In our article, we use the camera to send the input as video to our algorithms for crowd analysis.

CrowdNet Algorithm for Crowd Detection

CrowdNet is primarily an algorithm that uses two different variations of detecting people for the same image (Deep network algorithm and shallow network algorithm) to obtain the best possible accuracy. The first challenge CrowdNet aims to tackle with a hybrid algorithm is the difference in scaling as the distance between the camera and the person increases.

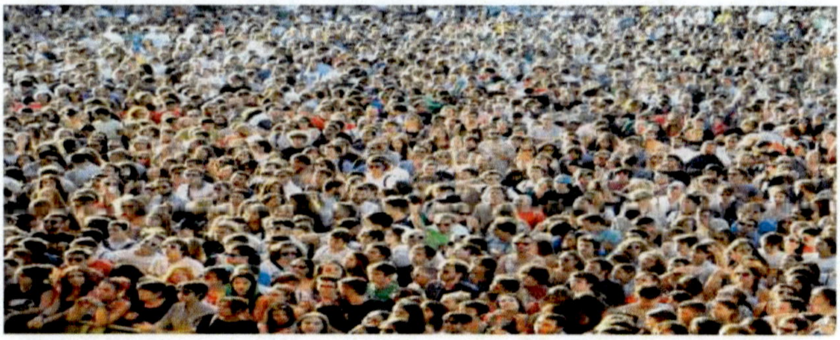

Fig. (2). Still of a crowd.

With reference from Fig. (**2**), If a person were to stand near the camera, he would scale much more prominent than he is. The same applies when the person is standing away from the camera, and he would scale small. Due to the same phenomenon, we can observe a long road converging at the furthest distance. However, they maintain the same width. When a densely populated image is given, we can only rely on a few pixels to detect a person. This creates a significant margin for error. This is the second challenge this algorithm aims to tackle. One body part always visible in the event of dense crowds is the head of the masses. This is a phenomenon CrowdNet takes huge advantage of.

YOLO Open CV Flow Model

Pre-recorded video is fed as an input to provide a replacement for real-time video input. Each frame is being analyzed using the YOLO object detection model, and then they are scanned to check for more than 5 people in one location. The detected people are enclosed by a bounding box. The ones standing very close are enclosed using red bounding boxes. The number of people detected from the video frame is sent to the online Ubidots platform. The data is then compared to a threshold value which is 5. When the number of people in a crowd exceeds 5, an alert is sent to using events on Ubidots through Telegram and Gmail. When the crowd is cleared, an alert message, informing that the crowd has been cleared, is also sent.

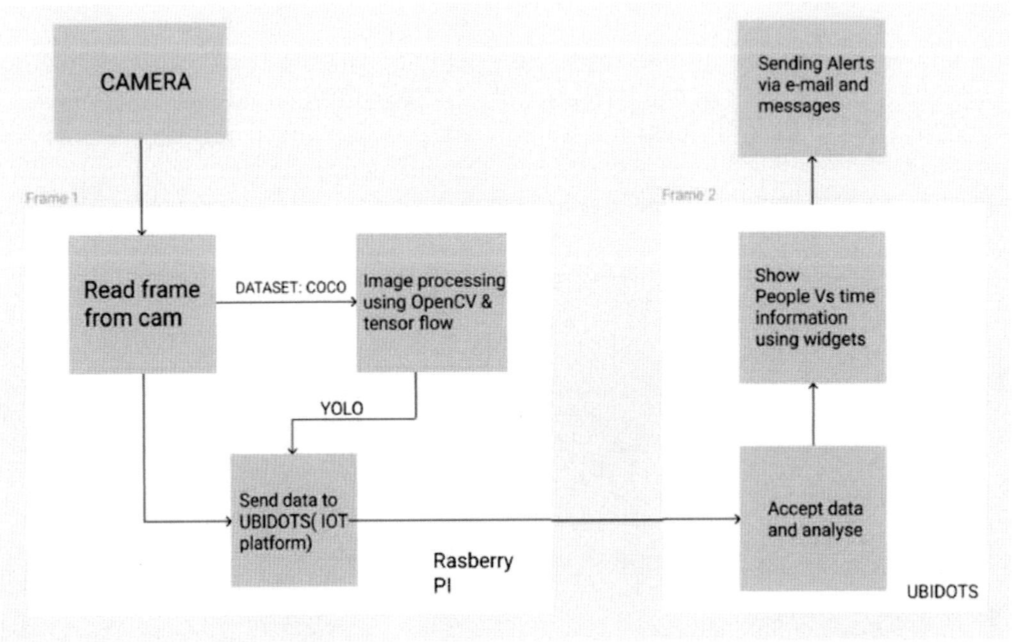

Fig. (3). Flow diagram of YOLO model.

All the required libraries such as TensorFlow and OpenCV are set up as the first step inside Raspberry Pi as represented in Fig. (**3**). The image width and height are set, and smaller resolutions can be used for a faster frame rate. The required camera module is selected as either Raspberry Pi or USB camera. The user is given the option to select the required camera module through argparse. The ssdlite_mobilenet_v2_coco_2018_05_09 contains the object detection module. This directory is defined as the next step to start with object detection. The TensorFlow files - frozen_inference_graph.pb,mscoco_label_map.pbtxt are loaded in accordance with the current working directory path. The .pf file - protobuf file contains all the graph definitions as well as the weight of the model. The .pb file cannot be trained; further is needed to run a trained model. Label and label maps are loaded along with the TensorFlow model into memory. Input and output tensors are defined, the input tensor is the image, and the output tensor is the object detection. The raw output is taken from a pi camera or USB camera and is passed as an input image for detection, and output indicates the number of people in the frame and violation of the rules - social distancing. This output, or the number of people detected in the video frame, is sent to the Online Ubidots platform as seen in Fig. (**5**). Using the VideoCapture() function of OpenCV, the pictures are taken every 5 seconds. Using the ret function, the frames are extracted, and then the resized frames are sent to Ubidots. Fig. (**4**) shows Ubidots offers various ways to set up the dashboard, which will allow the user to visualize the data easily and clearly. The chart widget is used to plot a graph between the crowd density and the time. The green and red boxes are the bounding boxes enclosing individuals. Furthermore, by applying the formula of euclidean, the distance between the centres of 2 bounding boxes is found. If the distance is less than the social distance that is to be maintained, the green bounding boxes turn red. Furthermore, they are accounted for as violations. Ubidots has a device that calculates and displays the violations by using the violation widget as shown in Figs. (**4** and **5**).

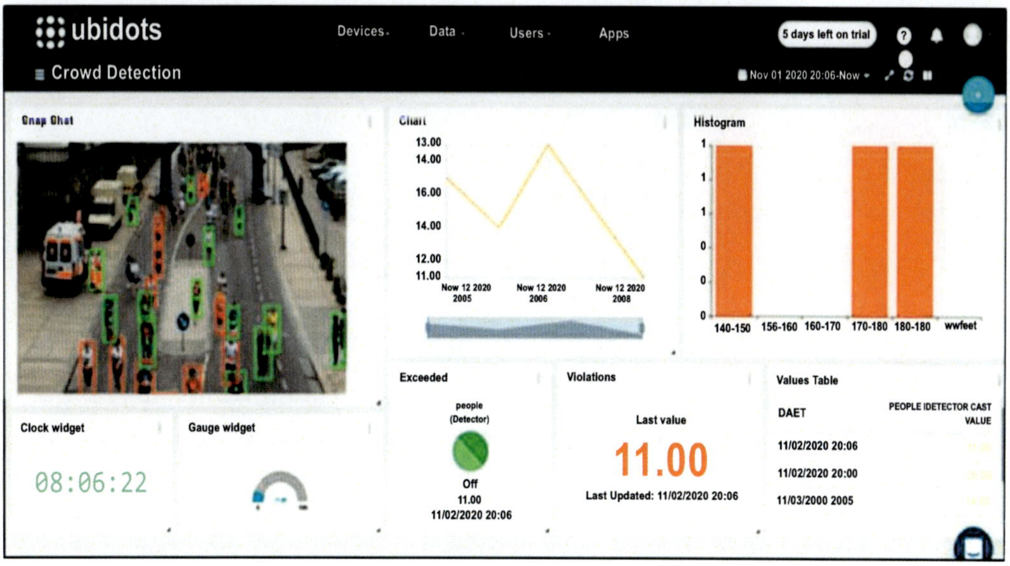

Fig. (4). People *vs.* time graph on UBIDOTS IoT platform.

The same result is depicted by using different widgets such as the Histogram or the values table, and a clock widget is also incorporated to show the time when the data was collected. Another feature that Ubidots offers is sending an alert *via* e-mail or a message whenever the threshold is crossed. Fig. (**6**) shows the automated message. This threshold value can be set or changed by us on the Ubidots.

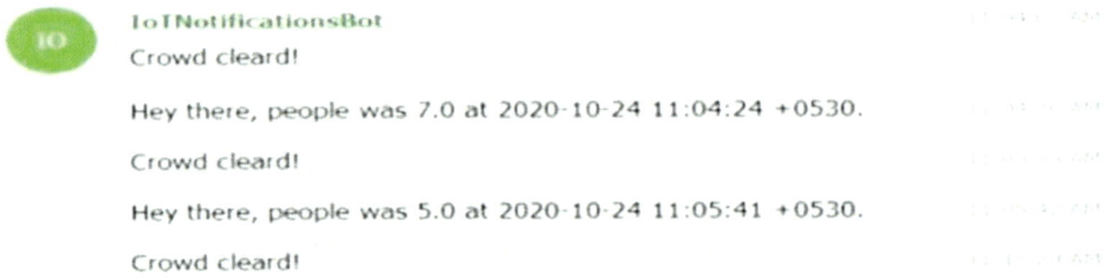

Fig. (5). E-mail crowd cleared notification sent by UBIDOTS.

A message is sent to the registered number when the threshold is crossed and even when the crowd is cleared.

Fig. (6). E-mail alert notification sent by UBIDOTS.

The same information is sent to the entered e-mail address as well as seen in Fig. (**6**).

Data Analytics for Collected Crowd Data Based on Location Tags

All the results are recorded into a .csv file in the backend through a python script. From Figs. (**7** to **10**), the CSV files contain fields such as Timestamp, Rule violated, area-id, city id, preferred, and date. When much data is accumulated over time, if an analysis had to be made, it would not be easy to analyze massive data. We made the following for data analytics; a spring boot application is made with java services such as jpa, getter setter methods to pull the data from a .csv file as shown in Fig. (**7**) and update it on the Postgres database shown in Fig. (**8**). Fig. (**9**) shows the docker run environment which the Apache Superset dashboard is running on. From the Postgres Database, the data is uploaded to Apache superset in Fig. (**10**). Hence when any query is applied in a superset, the entire data is fetched from the database and visualized for the user. This gives an effective way to visualize and also analyze data from the past, present, and future.

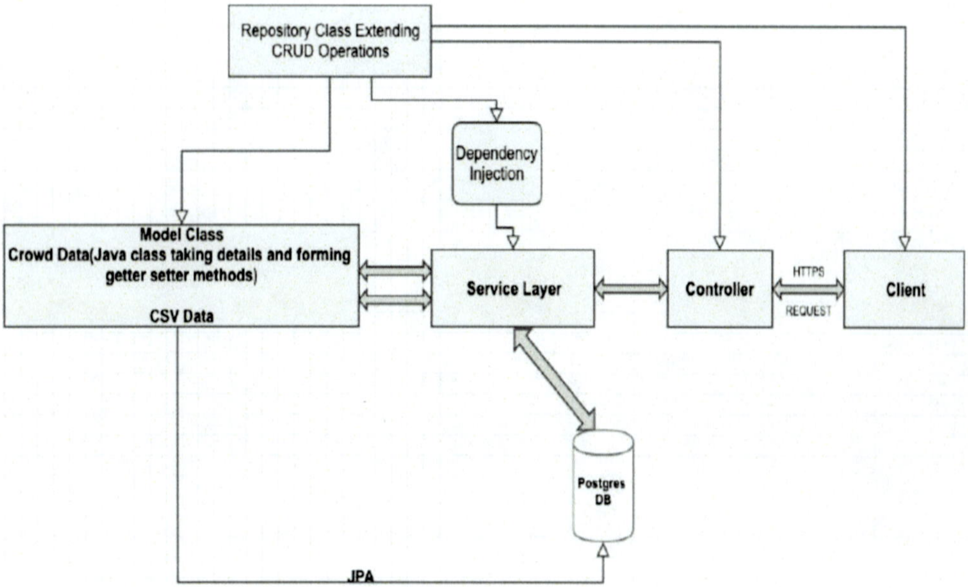

Fig. (7). Service layer architecture.

```
1 SELECT * FROM public.customer
2 ORDER BY id ASC
```

Date Output Explain Messages History

id [PK] integ	Time Stamp character varying (255)	rule_violated character varying (255)	from_area_id character varying (255)	from city_id character varying (255)	from date character varying (255
1	Time Stamp	rule_violated	from_area_id	from_city_id	from_date
2	1/1/2013 1:39	0	83	NULL	1/1/2013 2:00
3	1/1/2013 2:25	0	1010	NULL	1/1/2013 9:00
4	1/1/2013 3:08	0	1301	NULL	1/1/2013 3:30
5	1/1/2013 4:39	0	768	NULL	1/1/2013 5:45
6	1/1/2013 7:33	0	1363	NULL	1/1/2013 9:00
7	1/1/2013 8:01	0	1071	NULL	1/1/2013 22:30
8	1/1/2013 9:21	0	571	15	1/1/2013 9:45
9	1/1/2013 9:39	0	1192	NULL	1/1/2013 11:00
10	1/1/2013 9:44	0	448	NULL	1/1/2013 16:00
11	1/1/2013 9:49	0	516	NULL	1/1/2013 11:00
12	1/1/2013 9:55	0	156	NULL	1/1/2013 11:00
13	1/1/2013 9:59	0	455	NULL	1/1/2013 12:45
14	1/1/2013 10:18	0	1166	NULL	1/1/2013 12:30
15	1/1/2013 11:17	0	793	NULL	1/1/2013 12:45
16	1/1/2013 11:48	0	1063	NULL	1/1/2013 15:00
17	1/1/2013 11:52	0	1102	NULL	1/2/2013 2:00
18	1/1/2013 12:14	0	814	NULL	1/2/2013 0:30

Fig. (8). Postgres database output.

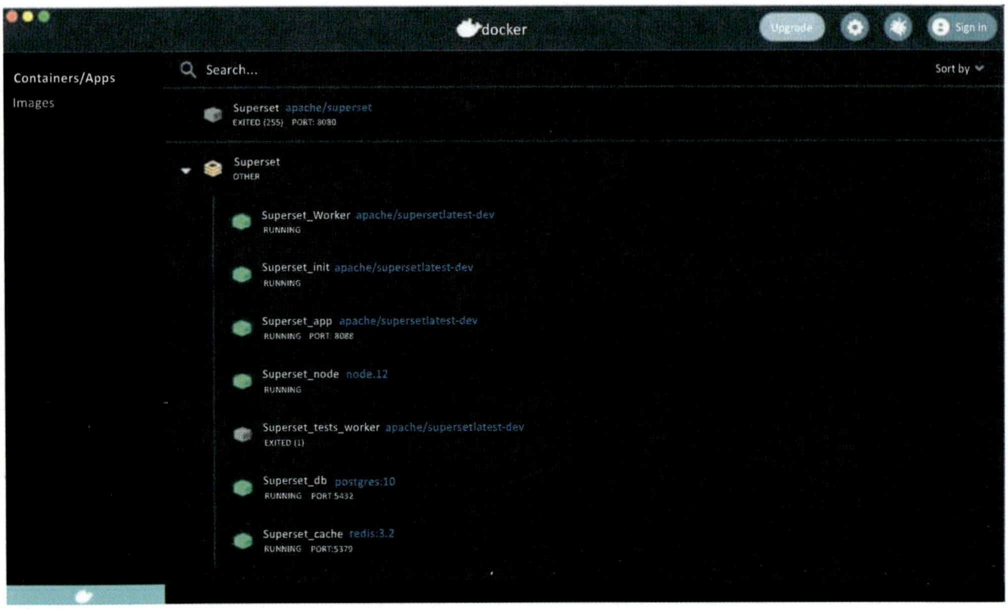

Fig. (9). Docker run time environment.

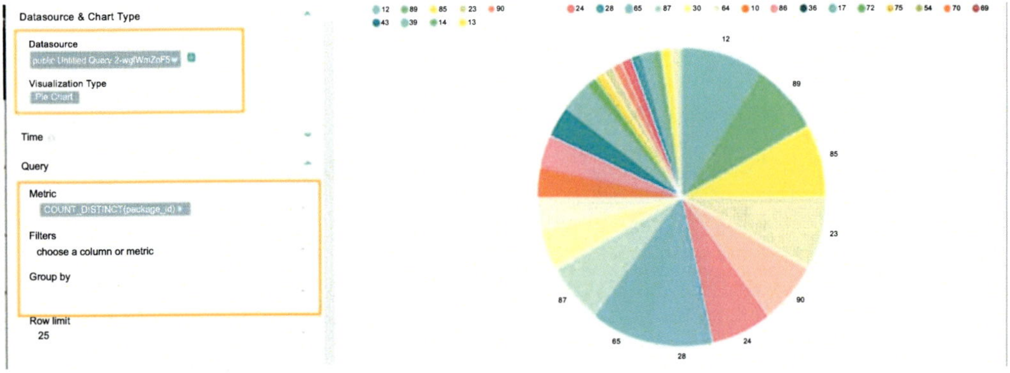

Fig. (10). Apache Superset dashboard showing people gathered in crowds at different location tags.

CrowdNet for Crowd Detection

To train a CNN algorithm, the algorithm is provided with a large number of datasets. The model is trained by keeping the gaussian kernel equal to one. The Gaussian kernel can be compared to a point in a graph. Although it is not strictly local, it can be called a semi-point. When the normalization or the area of integration is equal to one, the total divided by the quality of the gray level in the image is the same as when we blur the image with the Gaussian kernel. Preparing in the mentioned methods allows the CNN to learn faster when compared because the Gaussian kernel takes the head as a semi-point and does not pinpoint a single pixel. This method can help in making accurate predictions. On average, it takes 5 hours of training time for one fold in CrowdNet.

A point of difference that CrowdNet has over conventional CNN algorithms is that it can detect crowd density in a highly dense environment with relatively good accuracy. CrowdNet is trained on a deep convolutional network on the Deeplab version of Caffe (deep learning framework). CrowdNet uses a deep and shallow network depending upon the scenario as shown in Fig. (**11**). The Hardware used to train is the Titan X as the Graphical Processing Unit (GPU).

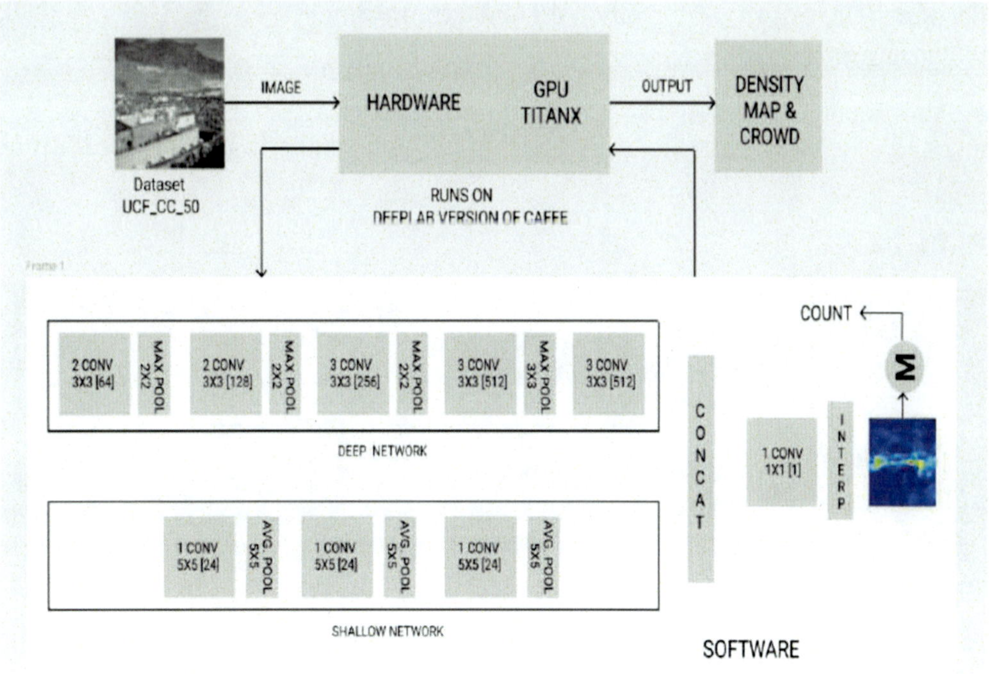

Fig. (11). CrowdNet model.

Caffe is a deep learning system that prioritizes versatility, speed, and modularity. Berkeley AI Research (BAIR) and group collaborators are working on it. During his Ph.D. at UC Berkeley, Yangqing Jia developed this prototype. DeepLab is a cutting-edge Caffe-based deep learning framework for semantic image segmentation. To begin, it uses atrous convolution to precisely monitor the resolution at which Deep Convolutional Neural Networks compute feature responses. Second, atrous spatial pyramid pooling is used to reliably segment artefacts at different scales using filters with different sampling rates and efficient fields of view. Finally, as post-processing, densely bound conditional random fields (CRF) are used.

With a learning rate of 1e-7 and momentum of 0.9, the system was trained *via* a Stochastic Gradient Descent (SGD) optimization method. The iterative method in stochastic gradient descent (often abbreviated SGD) is used to refine an objective function with appropriate smoothness characteristics. A five-fold cross-validation method was used to measure the performance of CrowdNet. The data frame is randomly divided five times, and each of these data frames contains ten images. One of the data frames is kept aside, and is used to validate the performance of the algorithm (CrowdNet). The other 40 data frame images are trained using the method shown earlier.

To experiment, a challenging UCF_CC_50 dataset is used [17]. The dataset contained a variety of images, ranging from religious gatherings to political rallies to concerts.

RESULTS

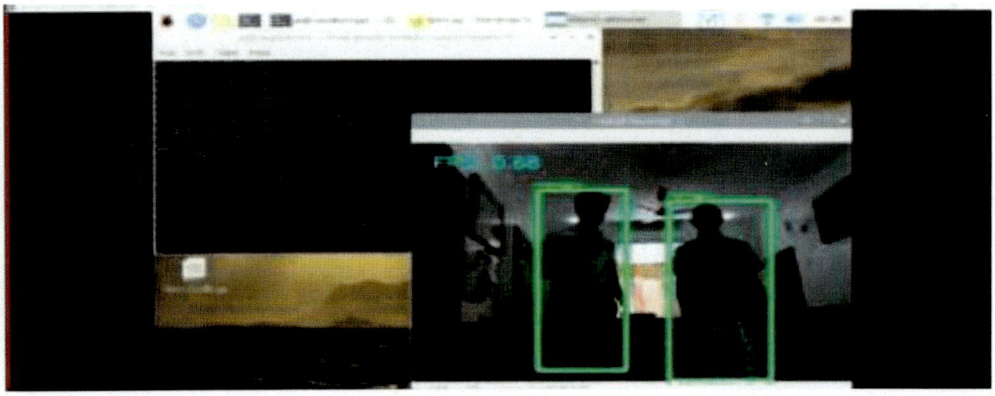

Fig. (12). Object detection using Raspberry Pi.

Fig. (**12**) shows an object detection of the Raspberry Pi Desktop. There are two windows; namely, the Terminal continuously shows whether people are detected, and if people are detected, then it shows the number of people—the Object Detector window, where the system takes in the information and processes it in real-time.

These are results from the CrowdNet as follows. Two images with a high-density count were fed into the system. The image is shown below. The dataset used was UCF_CC_50.

Table 1. Actual count *vs.* count estimated by Crowd Net.

-	Actual Count	Estimated
Image 1	1115	1143
Image 2	440	433

With the help of Fig. (**13**) and Table **1**, we can infer that the Actual count was 1115 and the estimated count was 1143. The count is overshoot by 28. In the second image, the actual count is 440, and the estimated count is 433. This prediction is very close to the actual value.

To assess the performance of CrowdNet, we can use the Mean Absolute Error (MAE). Mean Absolute Error is used to study the error between the measured and the actual value when working on the same image. Mean Absolute error (MAE) is an appropriate method when compared to root-mean-square-error (RMSE) since it is far more accurate in predicting the correct error [22].

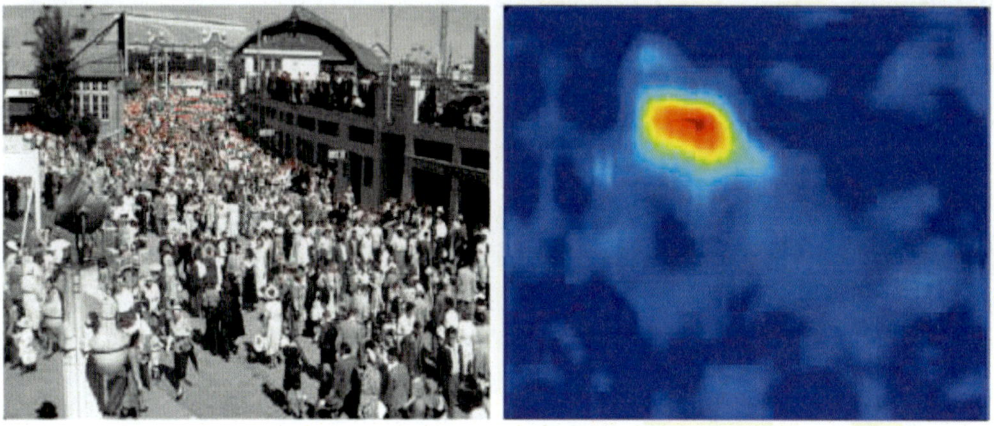

Fig. (13). CrowdNet detecting crowd density.

CONCLUSION AND FUTURE WORK

The proposed research work describes a thorough comparison between two models that can be used for efficient crowd detection and alert systems. These comparisons are based on specific essential metrics such as performance, material requirements, and processing power. The performance of both models can be compared based on the total number of people present in the crowd. CrowdNet performs better in high crowd density areas since it detects and counts the total number of heads in the image. At the same time, the YOLO model can be used when the cameras are placed in specific unusual orientations. It can detect the parts of human bodies; that is, it can detect a human presence by identifying their arms and legs. Another area of comparison can be the requirements. It can be concluded from the above paper that the material requirements for YOLO are considerably limited and therefore makes this a cheaper model. CrowdNet uses one of the most powerful GPUs (TITANX), which alone costs about Rs. 86,000. Thus when working for smaller crowds, YOLO is adopted. The processing power also makes a big difference when selecting which model to use. The power requirements of CrowdNet are very high since it uses the GPU TITAN X, which requires the user to download a considerable number of libraries and makes the entire model very heavy. The library requirements of YOLO are limited, and the functions used are also standard. The major constraint in the current implementation of crowd detection is that the current crowd counting methodologies are scene-explicit, as they are intended to work in the same environment utilized to prepare the system. Camera alignment can be used to accomplish scene invariance by scaling features suitably between perspectives. This empowers the framework to be sent on various preparing and testing sets. This is one of the prospective that was considered in our future implementation.

CONSENT FOR PUBLICATION

Not applicable.

CONFLICT OF INTEREST

The author declares no conflict of interest, financial or otherwise.

ACKNOWLEDGEMENT

Declared none.

REFERENCES

[1] D. Yang, "A Vision-based Social Distancing and Critical Density Detection System for COVID-19", *Research Gate.,* 2020. https://www.researchgate.net/profile/Ekim-Yurtsever/publication/342763051_A_Vision-based_Social_Distancing_and_Critical_Density_Detection_System_for_CO VID-19/links/5f08fbdc92851c52d628c8eb/A-Vision-based-Social-Distancing-and-Critical-Density-D-tection-System-for-COVID-19.pdf

[2] P. Sismananda, M. Abdurohman, and A.G. Putrada, "Performance Comparison of YOLO-Lite and YOLOV3 Using Raspberry Pi and MotionEyeOS", IEE Explore, 2020. https://ieeexplore.ieee.org/abstract/document/9166199

[3] A. Krizhevsky, "ImageNet classification with deep convolutional neural networks", 2017. Https://Dl.Acm.Org/Doi/10.1145/306538610.1145/3065386

[4] M.D. Chaudhari, and A.S. Ghotkar, "A Study on Crowd Detection and Density Analysis for Safety Control", *Int. J. Comput. Sci. Eng.,* vol. 6, no. 4, pp. 424-428, 2018. [http://dx.doi.org/10.26438/ijcse/v6i4.424428]

[5] N. Kumar, " An improved CNN framework for detecting and tracking human body in unconstraint environment", *ScienceDirect.,* 2020. https://linkinghub.elsevier.com/retrieve/pii/S0950705119305337 [http://dx.doi.org/10.1016/j.knosys.2019.105198]

[6] L. Boominathan, S.S.S. Kruthiventi, and R. Venkatesh Babu, "CrowdNet: A Deep Convolutional Network for Dense Crowd Counting", *Research Gate.,* 2016. https://www.researchgate.net/publication /306376987_CrowdNet_A_Deep_Convol [http://dx.doi.org/10.1145/2964284.2967300]

[7] G. Castellano, C. Castiello, C. Mencar, and G. Vessio, "Crowd Detection in Aerial Images Using Spatial Graphs and Fully-Convolutional Neural Networks", *IEEE Access,* vol. 8, pp. 64534-64544, 2020. [http://dx.doi.org/10.1109/ACCESS.2020.2984768]

[8] M.B. Shami, S. Maqbool, H. Sajid, Y. Ayaz, and S.C.S. Cheung, "People Counting in Dense Crowd Images Using Sparse Head Detections", *IEEE Trans. Circ. Syst. Video Tech.,* vol. 29, no. 9, pp. 2627-2636, 2019. [http://dx.doi.org/10.1109/TCSVT.2018.2803115]

[9] X. Ding, Z. Lin, F. He, and Y. Wang, *DEEPLY-RECURSIVE CONVOLUTIONAL NETWORK FOR CROWD COUNTING. Arxiv.Org.,* 2018. https://arxiv.org/pdf/1805.05633.pdf

[10] H. Reza Arkian, A. Diyanat, and A. Pourkhalilia, *MIST: Fog-based data analytics scheme with cost-efficient resource provisioning for IoT crowdsensing applications.,* 2017. https://linkinghub .elsevier.com/retrieve/pii/S1084804517300188

[11] D. Kong, D. Grey, and H. Tao, *Counting Pedestrians in Crowds Using Viewpoint Invariant Training.,* 2005. https://www.researchgate.net/publication/221260165_Counting_Pedestrians_in_ [http://dx.doi.org/10.5244/C.19.63]

[12] A. Bashir, and U. Izhar, *Compliance and Monitoring System for Businesses and Public Offices. MDPI.,* 2020. https://www.mdpi.com/2673-4591/2/1/14#cite

[13] N.I. Hassan, N.M. Tahir, F.H.K. Zaman, and H. Hashim, " People Detection System Using YOLOv3 Algorithm", In: *International Conference on Control System, Computing and Engineering (ICCSCE).* IEEE, 2020, pp. 131-136. [http://dx.doi.org/10.1109/ICCSCE50387.2020.9204925]

[14] F. Richter, *How many jobs were lost in 2020 due to COVID-19? World Economic Forum.,* 2021. https://www.weforum.org/agenda/2021/02/covid-employment-global-job-loss/

[15] A. Kandola, *Coronavirus cause: Origin and how it spreads.,* 2020. https://Www.Medicalnewstoday .Com/Articles/Coronavirus-Causes#transmissionhttps://www.medicalnewstoday.com /articles/coronavirus-causes#transmission

[16] M. Manfredi, and R. Vezzani, *Detection of static groups and crowds gathered in open spaces by texture classification.,* 2014. https://linkinghub.elsevier.com/retrieve/pii/S0167865513004248 [http://dx.doi.org/10.1016/j.patrec.2013.11.001]

[17] H. Idrees, I. Saleemi, C. Seibert, and M. Shah, "Multi-source multi-scale counting in extremely dense crowd images", In: *Conference on Computer Vision and Pattern Recognition.* IEEE, 2013. [http://dx.doi.org/10.1109/CVPR.2013.329]

[18] X. Wu, G. Liang, and K.K. Lee, *Crowd Density Estimation Using Texture Analysis and Learning.,* 2006. https://ieeexplore.ieee.org/document/4141867 [http://dx.doi.org/10.1109/ROBIO.2006.340379]

[19] R. Huang, J. Pedoeem, and C. Chen, "YOLO-LITE: A Real-Time Object Detection Algorithm

Optimized for Non-GPU Computers", In: *International Conference on Big Data (Big Data).* IEEE, 2018, pp. 2503-2510.
[http://dx.doi.org/10.1109/BigData.2018.8621865]

[20] S. Geethapriya, N. Duraimurugan, and S.P. Chokkalingam, "Real-Time Object Detection with YOLO", *Int. J. Eng. Adv. Technol.,* vol. 8, no. 3S, pp. 578-581, 2019. https://www.ijeat.org/wp-content/uploads/papers/v8i3S/C11240283S19.pdf [IJEAT].

[21] T. Ahmad, Y. Ma, M. Yahya, B. Ahmad, S. Nazir, and A. Haq, "Object Detection through Modified YOLO Neural Network", *Sci. Program.,* vol. 2020, pp. 1-10, 2020.
[http://dx.doi.org/10.1155/2020/8403262]

[22] C.J. Willmott, and K. Matsuura, "Advantages of the mean absolute error (MAE) over the root mean square error (RMSE) in assessing average model performance", *Clim. Res.,* vol. 30, no. 1, pp. 79-82, 2005. http://www.jstor.org/stable/24869236
[http://dx.doi.org/10.3354/cr030079]

CHAPTER 10

A Game-Based Neurorehabilitation Technology to Augment Motor Activity of Hemiparesis Patients

J. Sofia Bobby[1,*], **B. Raghul**[2] and **B. Priyanka**[3]

[1] *Department of Biomedical Engineering, Jerusalem College of Engineering, Chennai-100, India*

[2] *ZIFO R & D Solutions, Chennai, India*

[3] *VIT University, Chennai, India*

Abstract: Stroke recovery is the subsequent goal of stroke medicine. Rehabilitation and recovery research is exponentially increasing. However, several impediments impede the progress in the design of neurorehabilitation technology for stroke patient recovery. The conventional rehabilitation techniques for stroke recovery have some limitations like the absence of standardized terminology, poorly described methods, lack of consistent time frames and recovery biomarkers, reduced participation, and inappropriate measures to examine outcomes. Stroke recovery is challenging for many survivors. They require highly functioning and quick treatment accompanied by a gradual acceptance of brain improvement and human behavior. Therefore, there is an immediate need for neurorehabilitation technology to improve the quality of activities of daily life (ADLs) of those disabled. The method adopted is the design of neurorehabilitation technology using game-based systems that enhances the motor activities of hemiparesis patients.

Keywords: Arduino, Hemiparesis, Neurorehabilitation, Stroke, Visual feedback.

INTRODUCTION

Worldwide, Stroke is the second foremost reason for death and the third for disability. Low and middle-income countries are prone to stroke-associated deaths and disability-adapted life years. Stroke is the lack of oxygen to the brain cells due to the rupture or blockage of an artery. It is considered a risk factor for depression and dementia. Knowing the anatomy of the brain might assist in understanding the occurrence of the Stroke.

* **Corresponding author J. Sofia Bobby:** Department of Biomedical Engineering, Jerusalem College of Engineering, Chennai-100, India; E-mail: sofiabobbyj@Jerusalemengg.ac.in

Sivakumar R., Dimiter Velev, Basim Alhadidi, S. Vidhya, Sheeja V. Francis and B. Prabadevi (Eds.)

Anatomy and Physiology of Brain

The brain weighs almost three pounds. It controls all the body functions. It involves interpreting the information and integrating the core of the mind and soul. A few of the many functions of the brain are intelligence, creativity, emotion and memory. It comprises the cerebrum, cerebellum and brain stem Fig. (**1**) shows the anatomy of the brain.

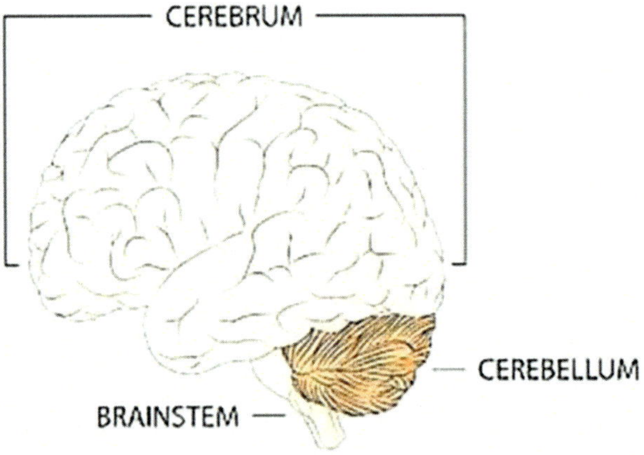

Fig. (1). Anatomy of the brain.

The cerebrum occupies the largest part of the brain. It comprises four individual lobes: the frontal, temporal, parietal and occipital. Each lobe posses varied functions, some of which may intersect.

Frontal Lobe

Motor function, problem-solving, spontaneity, memory, language, initiation, judgment, impulse control, and social and sexual behaviour.

Temporal Lobe

Memory, hearing, and understanding of speech and distinguishing between sounds and smells.

Parietal Lobe

Sensory comprehension, interpreting taste, touch, temperature, pain, movement and orientation.

Occipital Lobe

Visual stimuli.

The cerebrum, in the middle, can be divided into two parts. The left side of the brain, the left hemisphere, controls the right side of the body. The right side of the brain, the right hemisphere, controls the left side of the body. This provides a better understanding of why Stroke affects one side of the body. The lobes of the cerebrum is shown in Fig. (**2**).

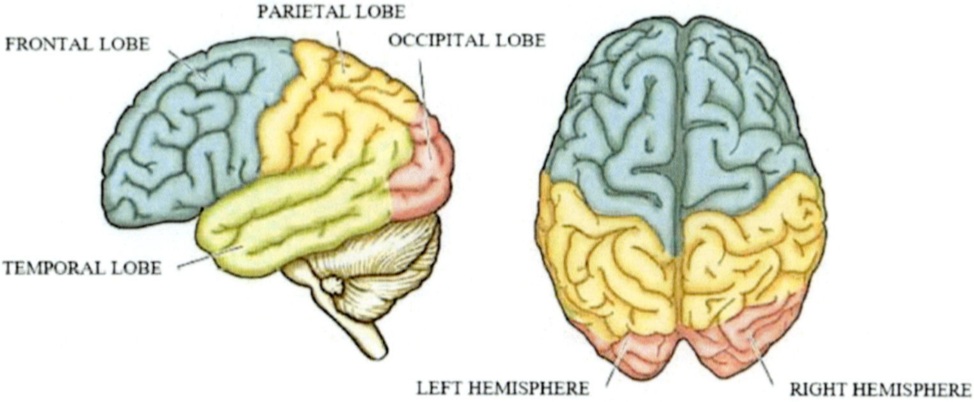

Fig. (2). Lobes of the cerebrum (Courtesy: sciencedirect.com).

The Cerebellum

The cerebellum resides behind the brainstem. The cerebellum modifies the movements controlled by the frontal lobe. It is responsible for fine motor movement, balance, and the brain's ability to determine position. Stroke occurring in this area may result in convulsive muscle movements.

The Brain Stem

The brain stem is otherwise known as Medulla Oblongata. It locates at the top of the spinal column. It regulates alertness, heart rate, blood pressure, and breathing. A stroke occurring in this area may disrupt breathing and result in sudden death.

Definition of Stroke

Sudden cessation of blood supply to the brain causes a stroke. An unexpected blockage in the artery (ischemic stroke) causes most of the strokes. Another stroke is due to the bleeding when a blood vessel bursts (hemorrhagic stroke). The region of the brain and the degree of damage determines the signs and symptoms of a stroke. The consequences of the stroke may be loss of sensation, weakness, or problems with seeing, speaking, and walking. The mortality rate for hemorrhagic stroke is seen as higher than for ischemic stroke.

Ischemic Stroke

Almost 87% of stroke cases report the stroke type as ischemic. It is caused due to blockage in an artery from a thrombus or clogged vessels due to atherosclerosis. In atherosclerosis, the inner diameter of the artery gets narrowed. It occurs due to the deposition of cholesterol plaques within the walls of the arteries (Fig. **3A**). Since the artery gets narrowed, blood flow is reduced, and as a result, the blood pressure increases to meet the body's demand.

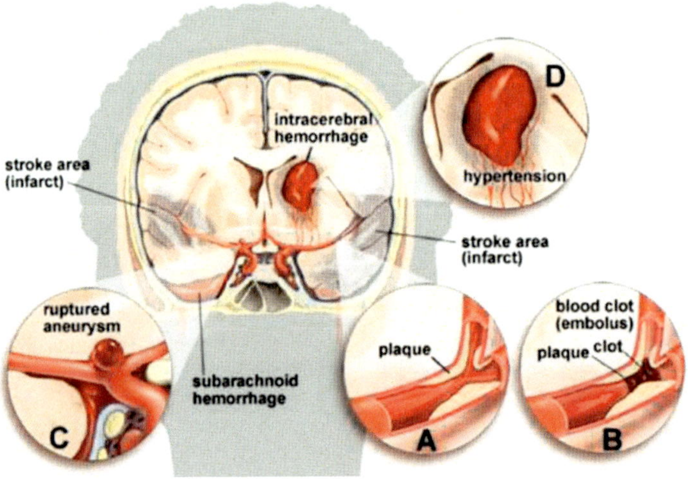

Fig. (3). A) Ischemic stroke; **B)** Embolic Stroke; **C)** Hemorrhagic Stroke and **D)** Intracerebral Stroke.

Embolic Stroke

It is caused due to the embolus forming as a clot bursts off from the artery and can travel down the bloodstream (Fig. **3B**). The emboli can travel down the bloodstream to block tiny arteries. They often originate from the heart.

Hemorrhagic Stroke

Hemorrhagic Stroke is less common. It is caused by the leaking or rupture of an artery either around or within the brain. It occurs when a blood vessel ruptures, releasing blood into the brain. It is also known as subarachnoid hemorrhage. It may be caused due to arteriovenous malformation (AVM), head trauma, or a ruptured aneurysm (Fig. **3C**). The mortality rate ranges from 30% to 40% and exceeds 50% for anticoagulant-related intracerebral hemorrhages [1].

Intracerebral Stroke

Intracerebral hemorrhage ICH is characterized by bleeding within the brain tissue itself. It is primarily caused by hypertension (Fig. **3D**). Hypertension is an elevation of blood pressure that may cause tiny arteries to burst inside the brain.

Symptoms

Stroke symptoms may occur alone or in combination and last a few minutes or several hours. The prevention and advancement in Stroke treatment are limited due to a lack of knowledge among the public. A high level of Stroke might follow even after the disappearance of symptoms of a stroke.

• One-sided sudden numbness or weakness of the arm, face or leg in the body.

• Speaking difficulty.

• One or double-sided low or blurred vision.

• Unexpected or inappropriate dizziness.

At times, strokes are followed by transient ischemic attacks, a mini-stroke lasting for many hours or a few minutes. This occurs due to a temporary blockage of the brain blood flow. However, it is restored later. The person becomes normal after its occurrence. Before a big stroke, many TIAs are possible to occur, which is a major warning.

Causes

The risk factors that cannot be altered are age, gender and race.

The risk factors that can be altered are high blood pressure (hypertension), smoking, weight, diabetes, TIA and heart disease.

Diagnosis

Initially, the doctor will try to get more details on current and earlier medications, associated problems, family history and symptoms. Then a physical exam is done along with information gathering from the patient, family members, or friends. Stroke is diagnosed *via* various procedures, including,

• **Lumbar Puncture -** It is done to detect blood in the cerebrospinal fluid in case of hemorrhagic Stroke. In this procedure, a hollow needle is inserted in the Spinal canal's subarachnoid space.

• **Computed Tomography (CT)** – It is done to study anatomical structures of the brain in case of both ischemic and hemorrhagic strokes. This is a non-invasive x-ray imaging technique.

• **Angiogram** - This is done to locate and determine an aneurysm in the brain in case of both ischemic and hemorrhagic strokes. It is an invasive procedure in which a catheter is inserted into an artery, and through the blood vessels, it reaches the brain. Also, a contrast dye is injected into the bloodstream to capture the X-ray images.

• **Magnetic Resonance Imaging (MRI) -** This is done to study a detailed view of soft tissues of the brain in case of both ischemic and hemorrhagic strokes.

Treatment and Recovery

Treatment

The therapy for both types (ischemic or hemorrhagic) of Stroke is different. In either case, the person must get to a hospital immediately for the treatments to work.

Ischemic stroke treatments can be divided into emergency treatments to reverse a blockage and preventive treatments to prevent Stroke.

Emergency procedures

• Clot buster drugs (tPA-tissue Plasminogen Activator)

• Clot retrieval devices

• Preventive procedures

• Blood thinners

• Angioplasty/stents

• Carotid endarterectomy

Haemorrhagic stroke treatment focuses on stopping the bleeding.

Recovery

Each person's mental and physical deficits are unique. Someone with a small stroke may experience only minor deficits, such as weakness of an arm or leg, while someone with a larger stroke may be left paralyzed on one side or lose his or her ability to speak. Some deficits may disappear over time with healing and therapy.

The recovery process is long, and regaining function may take months or years. Rehabilitation professionals can help set up a treatment plan and help loved ones understand the patient's needs for assistance with daily living activities. Some of the conditions during the recovery period are,

• **Aphasia,** caused by damage to the brain's language center, is a total or partial loss of the ability to understand or use words.

• **Apraxia** is the inability to control the muscles, making movements uncoordinated and jerky.

• **Dysarthria** is a loss of control over muscles in the face and mouth. A person's voice may sound slurred, muffled, or hoarse. The mouth may droop on one side of the face because of muscle weakness.

• **Dysphagia** is difficulty swallowing, making eating and drinking a challenge and choking a danger.

• **Paralysis** is a loss of muscle function and sensation in an area of the body.

• **Paresis** is a weakness of the muscles of the body. Improving posture, range of motion, and strength can help individuals regain control.

There are basically three types of paresis existing – Quadriparesis, Paraparesis and Hemiparesis, as shown in Fig. (**4**). We mainly focus on the Hemiparesis part, where the individual loses complete control on one side.

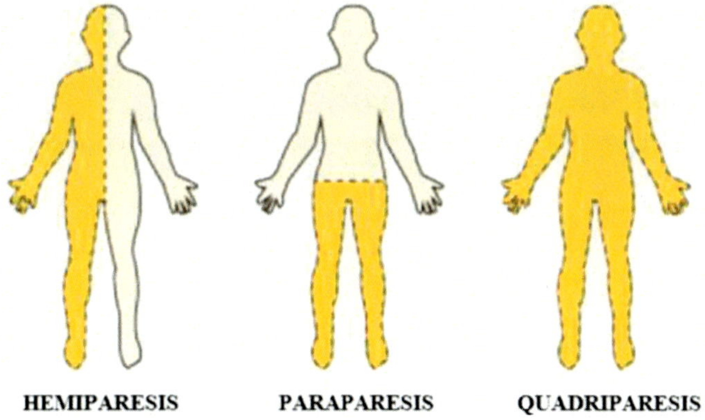

Fig. (4). Types of paresis (courtesy: Encyclopedia).

Existing Technology

Stroke patients with hemiparesis or hemiplegia may have difficulty with everyday activities such as walking or grasping objects [2]. The rehabilitation process for hemiparesis patients is a tedious process where the patients are engaged in doing a lot of exercises. Physical and occupational therapy help reverse disabilities caused by Stroke. By encouraging the use of the affected parts of the body through exercise, the patient can slowly relearn the ability to use them again. Recovery occurs through overcoming learned non-use, learning to use existing redundant neural pathways that do not include damaged brain tissue, and the development of new neural pathways through brain plasticity. This very demanding process can require hundreds of repeated motions every day to progress towards recovery. Therapy with repetitive exercises can provide the brain with sufficient stimuli to remodel itself and provide better motor control.

Some of the existing therapies are:

Therapeutic Rehabilitation Exercise

The massed practice of stroke rehabilitation exercises is the best way to improve movement, especially at home. By completing high repetition of physical therapy exercises, the brain can be rewired through neuroplasticity.

Music Therapy

Music helps enrich the environment, which has been shown to enhance sensory, social, cognitive, and motor activity. Music therapy for stroke patients helps stimulate multiple brain functions, including motor function and attention.

Constraint Induced Movement Therapy

CIMT is a superior method for combating learned non-use, a condition that occurs when mobility impairments continue to worsen after Stroke.

Robot-Based Rehabilitation

Essentially, robot-assisted therapy utilizes special machines that help patients complete their rehab exercises. This helps patients complete more repetitions than they could on their own, which helps the brain recover faster.

Mirror Therapy

Mirror therapy for stroke patients, can help improve hand mobility “tricking” the brain into believing that the non-affected hand is moved. This stroke rehabilitation technique is so powerful that it often plays a central role in the most inspiring hand paralysis recovery stories.

Magnetic Brain Stimulation

During magnetic brain stimulation, wires are placed on the scalp, and current stimulation is sent to the brain. The stimulation helps excite the damaged parts of the brain and boost recovery. Both acute and chronic stroke patients can benefit from brain stimulation.

Problems with Conventional Technology

However, research suggests that most stroke survivors do not perform sufficientrepetitionstomakeprogresstowardsrecoveryandthatmoststroke survivors need to exercise by themselves at home to achieve enough repetitions. Repeating the same movements hundreds of times can be far from exciting. These rehabilitation exercises make them get tired easily and need the help of other people. It can be also noted that the robotics technologies are more expensive to accommodate. The perceptive view of the patient also indicates the mind to finish the exercises soon or the thought of the remaining exercises. Thus, the main problems encountered can be concluded as Vigorous exercise, Other support, Cost and Lack of interest.

The explosion of knowledge about the stroke-damaged brain must be incorporated into our collective thinking about the nature and delivery of rehabilitation and restorative therapies [3]. Variable methodological quality of animal studies [4], poorly defined interventions [5], and lack of agreed methods for developing, monitoring, evaluating and reporting interventions limit translation of research into evidence-based therapies [6]. Furthermore, patient descriptions are not standardized,recoverybiomarkersarenotwelldefined [7], and there is a lack of agreed time-points or measures to examine outcomes in rehabilitation and recovery trials [8].

It is observed that 10 percent of stroke victims make a nearly complete recovery, 10 percent require long-term care following a stroke, and 15 percent die shortly after a stroke, meaning that 65 percent of stroke patients require some level of rehabilitative therapy [9-13]. Rehabilitation is the process of recovering the existing skills of an injured or ill person so as to regain his/her maximum independence and function in normal life or as near normal manner as possible. The goal is to decrease long-term disability by designing a motivational game-based therapy based on inexpensive independent therapy.

Objective

Based on the overview of the potential use of controllers in the assessment of Rehabilitation, we propose a classification of these devices, and specify requirements for these technologies to be useful for the assessment of balance. This paper focuses on rehabilitation in stroke and hemiparesis, increasing the level of involvement of the patient. The games are specifically developed to perform exercises and to increase their involvement which in turn increase their Motor activity. We finalize by highlighting current challenges and recommendations for the adoption of gaming technology in clinical assessment of motor activity.

The main objective is to design a game-based neurorehabilitation technology for improving the quality of ADLs of hemiparesis patient by improving the motor activities with complete muscle recruitment.

HISTORY OF NEUROREHABILITATION

Neurorehabilitation interventions have exploded since the year 2000, in parallel with a shift in the paradigm of neurologic care. In the mid-20th century, we turned away from the assumption that the effect of a brain injury such as a stroke on function, activity, and participation is permanent and became increasingly aware of the brain's regenerative potential, as well as dynamic brain reorganization, months and even many years later. Neurorehabilitation scientists pushed for translational research to define the permissive conditions under which optimal brain change and recovery occurs, apparently requiring controlled, intensive stimulation of impaired brain networks.

Historical Perspectives

Knowing the history of physical therapy practice lets us reflect on transformation and development in clinical practice and to sense more comfortable with the idea that clinical practice must acknowledge and adapt as new scientific knowledge arises. The history of neurological physical therapy explains the process of change. Early in the 20th century, practitioners used corrective exercise and muscle re-education, the latter involving exercises directed at individual muscles. The understanding that clinicians implemented in their practice revealed an early focus on structural anatomy and principles of exercise. Many of the people receiving physical therapy were selves with muscle weakness and paralysis from poliomyelitis. This importance was to shift as the numbers of people acquiring poliomyelit is steadily diminished with new preventive therapies. Following the second world war, an inrush of young adults with acute brain injury sustained drive the development of new therapies.

Origins of the Neurofacilitation Approaches

In the 1950s, a major conceptual change in neurological physical therapy was apparent as the neurophysiological or neurofacilitation approaches were developed. The focus turned from the muscle to non-muscle elements. Methods were directed fundamentally at the nervous system with movement promoted by stimulation of the nervous system. Significant influences were the work of the Bobaths, in Bobath Therapy or Neurodevelopmental Therapy (NDT), and of Kabat, Knott, and Voss, whose methods of 11 movement facilitation were referred to as Proprioceptive Neuromuscular Facilitation (PNF). Other therapists also produced their ideas for therapy around this time, including Rood, Ayres, and Brunnstrom. These therapy advances are often referred to as eponymous as they were named after their originators. Although the originators had diverse and sometimes contradictory approaches, their methods revealed their interpretations of early neurophysiological writings with experimental models, including stimulus-response mechanisms, many of them based on animal models. Therapeutic methods are concentrated on promoting movement by afferent stimulation, specifically of muscle and joint proprioceptors and tactile receptors. Their methods were based on concepts of the restorative effects of encouraging developmental movement patterns and highlighted postural stability and normal movement patterns. The Bobaths supported the view that the normalizing of muscle tone by inhibiting spasticity (abnormal postural tone) should occur before more normal movement could be facilitated. They held the opinion that movements requiring effort would increase spasticity and should therefore be avoided. Interestingly, these approaches paid little recognition to advancements in neuroscience, including those related to the context-dependent nature of the movement.

Developments in the 1980s

The above therapeutic methods, particularly those of Bobath, Knott, and Voss, dominated the second half of the 20th century and are still extensively used. However, there were newer improvements during this time, as physiotherapists and others who had access to the scientific literature sought ways of transferring new scientific findings to clinical practice. These advancements took advantage of experimental work that focused on how humans obtain skills in movement or motor learning, muscle biology and muscle adaptability, and psychology. These improvements exhibited to a large degree the growing opportunity for physiotherapists to register in postgraduate courses, thereby increasing research skills and involvement in the accelerated study of specific scientific fields. Not surprisingly, they saw the clinical associations. The initial efforts at improving therapy methods to enhance functional movement were largely inductive, and this may have been somewhat due to the lack of a relevant scientific body of information on human 12 movement from which clinical relationships could be more deductively derived. Over the last few decades, however, technological improvements together with shifts in the conceptualization of how the human nervous system might function to perform a skilled movement, have been presenting a growing amount of movement-related research, in the fields of biomechanics and neuroscience, in particular, that has visible significance to clinical practice. Technological developments in motion analysis and electromyography (EMG) have enabled studies of actions such as walking, standing up and reaching to pick up an object that demonstrate the kinematic sand kinetic so feach action,including the specific postural adjustments. New brain imaging methods enable an examination of organizational changes occurring within the brain itself and of the experiences that might drive them, particularly the effects of patterns of use and learning.

The increase in clinically relevant research findings related to movement therefore made possible the development of neurological rehabilitation by a more deductive process. Clinical implications were derived from a theoretical science base, and new clinical methods were developed and tested. As an example, for the action of sit-to-stand, there is now a rational bio mechanical model that forms the basis for standardized guide lines for training this action. This model has also provided methods for measuring performance and an increased focus on clinical research is enabling us to test the efficacy of interventions.

Five Main Approaches

Here, we summarize 5 treatments to rehabilitate motor and cognitive recovery based on behavioral or non-invasive physiologic stimulation (using magnetic fields or electricity). They have been explored primarily in stroke rehabilitation but are also potentially useful after brain trauma and in other neurologic conditions (*e.g.*, spinal cord injury, multiple sclerosis).

Constraint-Induced Movement Therapy

Constraint-induced movement therapy (CIMT) for upper extremity paresis may be a prototypical example of translational neurorehabilitation. Intensive, experience-based, repetitive motor training of a paretic limb was first used in stroke survivors in the 1980s, based on the observation of "learned non-use" in monkeys with a deafferented limb but intact motor capability.Competent, symme tric movements were restored by immobilizing the unaffected for elimb. Thus, during CIMT administration, stroke survivors may wear a mitt on the unaffected hand during most waking hours to reinforce paretic arm use, and perform task-specific, repetitive movement shaping during 2 weeks of long daily sessions (3 – 6 hours).

A multisite CIMT study in chronic Stroke, the EXCITE trial, yields good results at time points 3–9 months and 15–21 months poststroke—later than most patients are eligible for conventional therapy. The participants were relatively mildly affected stroke survivors who had some ability to extend the wrist, thumb, or fingers and were able to stand unassisted for at least 2 minutes. The treatment is theoretically appealing: it may provide massed practice of functional movement in a paretic limb; the intensive practice, rather than the constraint, appears to support the CIMT treatment effect on brain reorganization. Since the main cost of treatment is therapist training, it is low risk and feasible for many clinical environments, but unfortunately third-party payers may not accept a daily treatment plan, even with 2 weeks duration. Also, studies indicate patients must have some preserved movement to improve. A "transfer package" therapeutic contract may aid with patient commitment and engagement to obtain best treatment results.

Weight-Supported Treadmill Training

Weight-supported treadmill walking, an intensive, experience-dependent functional movement training, is sometimes conceptually grouped with CIMT. Patients wear a supportive harness for this labor-intensive therapy, usually requiring a technician stationed at each leg to assist in leg advancement at a minimal walking speed. A third therapist/technician may be needed on the treadmill with the patient, to assist in trunk movements and balance. Although a recent study, the LEAPS trial, comparing treadmill-based training to home-based exercise showed no definite benefit of this approach on gait speed, walking ability, and balance control, some researchers still urge that we investigate whether stroke survivors, vulnerable to the ill effects of a sedentary lifestyle, may benefit from upright aerobic training with respect to general health (insulin resistance), bone mass, or psychological well-being.

Constraint-Induced Language Therapy

It is therapeutic effects of motor training on language recovery.

Taking a motor rehabilitation approach to a cognitive function such as language might seem odd. Traditionally, training gestures or movements in a communication program would be viewed as a way to avoid working on speech intensively—a "compensatory" rather than "experience-based" approach. However, it is possible that some treatments might support a function indirectly, an effect called "vicariation." "Vicariative" interventions may activate a neural system closely interacting with the stroke-impaired network so that both neural systems are functionally active during the treatment. Left brain stimulation and arm training after left brain stroke also resulted in language improvement. One explanation may be that movement training stimulates interrelated left-brain networks and supports both language and purposive arm/hand use.

Prism Adaptation Training For Spatial Neglect

Pathologically asymmetric reporting, response, or orienting to contralesional stimuli, causing functional disability (spatial neglect), affects >50% of acute stroke survivors, adversely affects recovery, and is associated with higher in-hospital and posthospital care expense. Spatial neglect treatments primarily addressed visual dysfunction, even though neuroscientists tell us that, distinct from visual-spatial errors, people with spatial neglect may make disabling, body-based, motor-exploratory spatial errors. Studies using a visual approach probably recruited subjects and assessed outcomes in ways that stack the deck against detecting improvements in spatial motor function. This translational block between neuroscience and clinical research may have confused clinicians. This may explain why neglect treatments reported to result in functional benefit are still not widely used.

Training sessions are brief (15–30 minutes); prisms are worn only during training, leaving the rest of the day free for other activities or rehabilitation. After training, with the lenses removed, participants typically demonstrate immediate after effects. Movements in the opposite direction (leftward). In stroke survivors with neglect, aftereffects may persist longer than in healthy controls, and improved leftward spatial motor "aiming" may generalize to improved daily life function. Dramatic improvements after PAT have been reported in some patients, who started self-ambulating in a wheelchair for navigation or gained new ability to self-dress after receiving PAT.

Transcranial Magnetic Stimulation

Transcranial magnetic stimulation (TMS) is a non-invasive method to stimulate the human brain; TMS has a role in evaluation of neurophysiology and diagnosis of many neurologic conditions. It is also emerging as a neuromodulating modality of great potential in debilitating psychiatric and neurologic disorders, although further studies are needed to support these preliminary findings.

A brief, strong magnetic field created by an electric current circulating within a coil on the scalp penetrates the skull and induces electrical current that can depolarize neurons and axons. Since TMS was first introduced in 1985, it has been used for clinical neurophysiology, intraoperative monitoring, and therapeutic purposes in a wide spectrum of neurologic and psychiatric conditions. As a diagnostic tool, TMS is primarily used for evaluation of cortical motor areas and motor pathways. Standard TMS methods of evaluation include assessing the motor threshold of the motor evoked potential (MEP; lowest stimulation intensity able to evoke MEP of minimal size) and central motor conduction time. Absent or low MEP suggests a loss of neurons or axons, and prolonged central conduction time may reflect demyelination of central motor pathway or loss of large fibres. However, clinical use of these methods is limited due to their complexity.

Research demonstrated that the excitatory or inhibitory effect of TMS on cortical excitability may persist when trains of repetitive TMS (rTMS) are deliveredovercorticalareas.TheeffectofrTMSoncorticalexcitabilitymay depend on the frequency of stimulation: downregulation may follow low- frequency rTMS (*e.g.*, 1 Hz) and excitation, high-frequency rTMS (*e.g.*, 10 Hz).There are some promising results using rTMS as an add-on therapy in a number of neurologic and psychiatric disorders characterized by dysfunction of distinct brain networks, including Stroke, tinnitus, chronic pain, and posttraumatic stress disorders. However, in United States, the only US Food and Drug Administration– approved indication of rTMS application is single- drug resistant unipolar depression. Further clinical trials are needed to support most claims of therapeutic utility of rTMS in many conditions.

A recent publication summarized safety precautions, ethical considerations, and application guidelines from a consensus conference for application of TMS in research and clinical settings. Although medical experience with the technique has in many ways been satisfactory, absolute contraindications for TMS use include the presence of metallic hardware in close contact to the discharging coil (such as cochlear implants, implanted brain electrodes, medical pumps). TMS use is also generally avoided in persons with a history of epilepsy, tumoral or infectious lesions of the brain, sleep deprivation, alcoholism, pregnancy, or severe heart disease. In general, an acceptable safety profile of TMS is well supported by the literature, although it is essential for TMS applicants to be familiar with potential side effects for safe, well-tolerated application (headache, syncope, seizure, hearing loss, magnetic induction of a metal or paramagnetic object, *etc.*).

HARDWARE AND SOFTWARE

The three main hardware's used are Arduino UNO board, an accelerometer and capacitive touch electrodes. These hardware's are integrated through two software's namely Arduino and Unity.

Hardware

The hardware's used are Arduino microcontroller, an accelerometer and capacitive touch electrodes. The description of all the hardware used is given below.

Arduino UNOBoard

The Arduino Uno is an open-source microcontroller board. It consists of a Microchip ATmega328P microcontroller. The board is equipped with 14 digital input/output pins and 6 analog input/output pins and is programmable *via* a type B USB cable using Arduino IDE. The function of each pin is shown in Table **1** and Arduino pin configuration is shown in Fig. (**5**). The power source can either be a USB cable or an external 9v battery. The ATmega328 is pre-programmed with a bootloader hence allow the uploading of new code without the use of an external hardware programmer.

Table 1. Arduino pin functions.

Pin Category	Pin Name	Details
Power	Vin, 3.3V, 5V, GND	Vin: Input voltage to Arduino when using an external power source. 5V: Regulated power supply used to power microcontroller and other components. 3.3V: 3.3V supply generated by on-board voltage regulator. GND: ground pins.
Reset	Reset	Resets the microcontroller.
Analog Pins	A0 – A5	Can be used as input or output pins in the range of 0-5V.
Digital Pins	0 - 13	Can be used as input or output pins.
Serial	0 (Rx), 1 (Tx)	Used to receive and transmit TTL serial data.
External Interrupts	2, 3	To trigger an interrupt.
PWM	3, 5, 6, 9, 11	Provides 8-bit PWM output.
SPI	10 (SS) 11 (MOSI) 12 (MISO) 13 (SCK)	Used for SPI communication.
Inbuilt LED	13	To turn on the inbuilt LED.
TWI	A4 (SDA), A5 (SCA)	Used for TWI communication.
AREF	AREF	To provide reference voltage for input voltage.

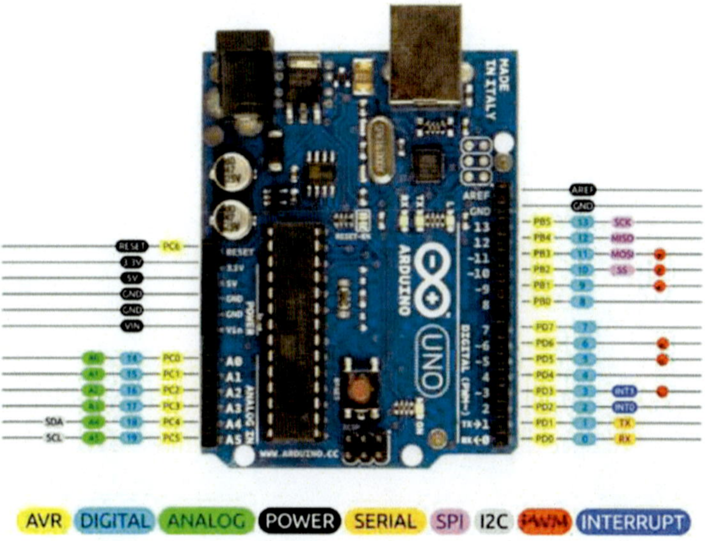

Fig. (5). Arduino pin configuration (Courtesy: Arduino.com).

The Arduino board technical specification are given in Table **2**,

Table 2. Arduino technical specifications.

Microcontroller	ATmega328P: 8-bit AVR family microcontroller
Operating Voltage	5V
Recommended Input Voltage	7-12V
Input Voltage Limits	6-20V
Analog Input Pins	6 (A0 – A5)
Digital I/O Pins	14 (Out of which 6 provide PWM output)
DC Current on I/O Pins	40 mA
DC Current on 3.3V Pin	50 mA
Flash Memory	32 KB (0.5 KB is used for Bootloader)
SRAM	2 KB
EEPROM	1 KB
Frequency (Clock Speed)	16 MHz

Sensor

Based upon the exercise (the exercises to augment motor activity of hemiparesis patients are described briefly in chapter) to be performed the sensors used in this project are:

i. Accelerometer (Palm up and down and Wrist bent movement) and

ii. Capacitive touch electrodes (Finger curl)

Accelerometer

The ADXL335 is a small, low-power, thin, 3-axis accelerometer. It is available in a small, low-profile,16-lead, plastic lead frame chip scale package (LFCSP_LQ) shown in Fig. (**6**) and pin descriptions are shown in Table **3**. It can measure the static acceleration of gravity in tilt-sensing and also dynamic acceleration from motion, vibration, or shock. It measures acceleration with a minimum full-scale range of ±3 g. Based on the application, the user can select the bandwidth with a range of 0.5 Hz to 1600 Hz for the X and Y axes, and a range of 0.5 Hz to 550 Hz for the Z-axis.

Table 3. ADXL335 pin descriptions.

Pin Name	Description
VCC	The V_{cc} pin powers the module, typically with +5V
GND	Power Supply Ground
X	X-axis Analog Output Pin
Y	Y-axis Analog Output Pin
Z	Z-axis Analog Output Pin
ST	Self-Test Pin. This pin controls the Self-Test feature.

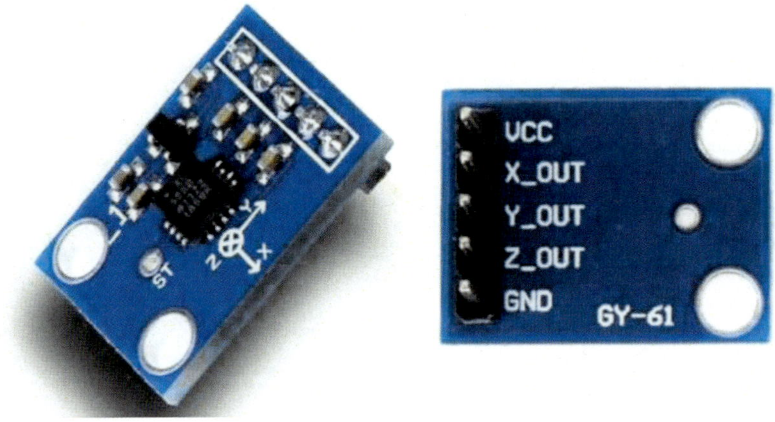

Fig. (6). ADXL335 (Courtesy: Wikipedia – Arduino).

Capacitive Touch Electrodes

The working principle of capacitive sensors is by the change of capacitance, the finger touching near the electrode. The change is too small to detect and hence challenging. The ability of the electrode to pick up the signal from the finger affects the overall performance significantly. The electric field projected from the transducer polarizes the object. In turn, the polarized charge attracts more charges from the source to join the transducer. An increase in charge storage means an increase in capacitance. This is how an external object increases the capacitance of the transducer. The Arduino pins are connected to a capacitive sensor. These pins can now sense the electrical capacitance of the human body. Now when the sensor is touched it produces output. The sensor setup requires a piece of copper conductive foil tape on the end and, a medium to high resistor, and a piece of wire as shown in Fig. (**7**).

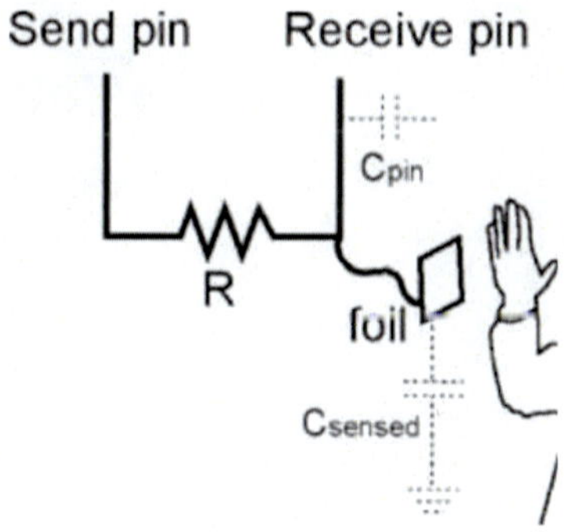

Fig. (7). Capacitive touch sensor circuit (Courtesy: Wikipedia).

When the sensor is more sensitive, it starts sensing the body inches away from the sensor. So, with a high resistor, it acts as a proximity sensor. The sensor designed with the help of copper conductive foil tape on the end is shown in Fig. (**8**).

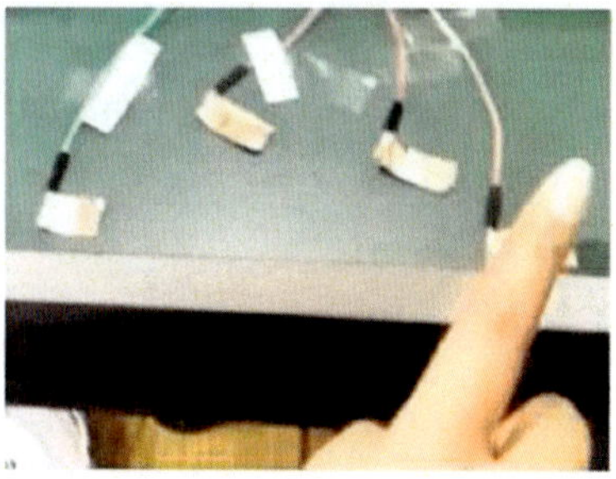

Fig. (8). Capacitive touch sensor setup.

Hand Glove Model

The main hardware component for this entire project is the hand gloves shown in Fig. (**9**). The hand gloves along with the sensors integrated forms the hand glove model. The sensors used are accelerometer and capacitive touch sensor. This project requires two types of Hand glove model based on its feasibility for the hemiparesis patient to perform exercises. The two types of hand glove model and their supporting exercises are given below:

Type 1: Palm up and down and wrist bent movement

Type 2: Finger curl

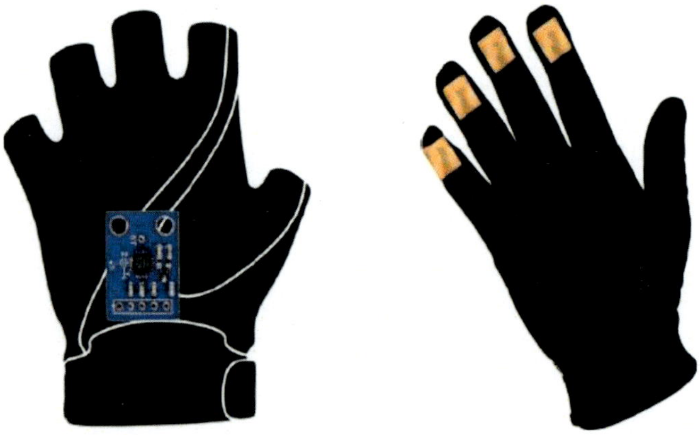

Fig. (9). Hand glove model: Type 1 (left); Type 2 (right).

Software

The software's used to build up this project are Arduino and Unity.

The description of all the software used is given below.

Arduino

The Arduino is an open-source platform. Its hardware and software are easy to use. The Arduino board can be programmed by a set of instructions, to perform a set of operations. To perform these operations, Arduino programming language and Arduino Software IDE are necessary. The software is open-source that enables the user to learn independently. The Arduino IDE has a text editor to write the code. It also contains a message area, a text console, a toolbar with buttons for common functions and, a series of menus. To communicate and upload the programs onto the board, the software has to be connected with the hardware. The programs are called sketches and are written in the text editor. The sketches are then saved with the file extension .ino. Cutting, pasting, searching, and replacing the text are some features found in the text editor. Feedback related to saving, exporting, and display errors can be seen in the message area. The console presents the text output and a window present at the bottom right-hand corner displays the configured board and serial port. The buttons present in the toolbar enable the user to create, open, save, verify, and upload sketches and also to open the serial monitor. The menu bar consists of file, edit, sketch, tools, and help. The Arduino IDE screen is given in Fig. (**10**) and Arduino Command symbols are shown in Table **4**.

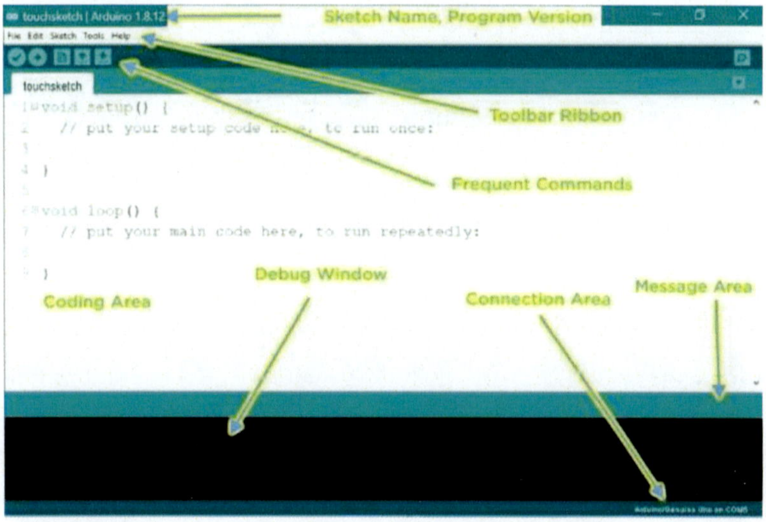

Fig. (10). Arduino screen.

Unity

Unity is a user-friendly development environment and a powerful cross-platform 3D engine (Fig. **11**). It interests beginners and experts to create applications and 3D games for consoles, web, desktop, and mobile. Unity is a perfect 3D environment. It includes functions: creating menus, laying out levels, doing animation, writing scripts, and organizing projects. It owns a well-organized user interface. The panels are customizable by drag and drop operation. The sections of the Unity game engine are:

• Project panel - The assets within the project are stored. The assets get displayed when imported.

• Hierarchy panel - Assets are organized in the hierarchy panel. To add the assets from the project panel into the current scene, they are dragged into the hierarchy panel.

• Inspector panel - A selected asset attribute can be inspected and adjusted through the inspector panel. The designer can control its position, rotation, the influence of gravity, and the casting of shadows.

• Scene panel - The scene panel is a 3D viewport. By moving the assets around the 3D space, they can be physically arranged in it.

• Assets - Any resources used in the games such as 3D models, materials, textures, audio, scripts, and fonts, *etc.* are known as assets. Unity can't create many of the assets except few objects such as cubes and spheres. Such assets are imported by creating them externally using 3D modelling applications and painting tools.

• Scripts - In Unity, scripts are known as behaviours. Scripts allow the designer to make the assets interactive. To a single object, multiple scripts can be attached. Unity scripts can be written using 3 different languages such as Unity Script, C#, and Boo. Unity Script resembles JavaScript and ActionScript, C# resembles Java, and Boo resembles Python.

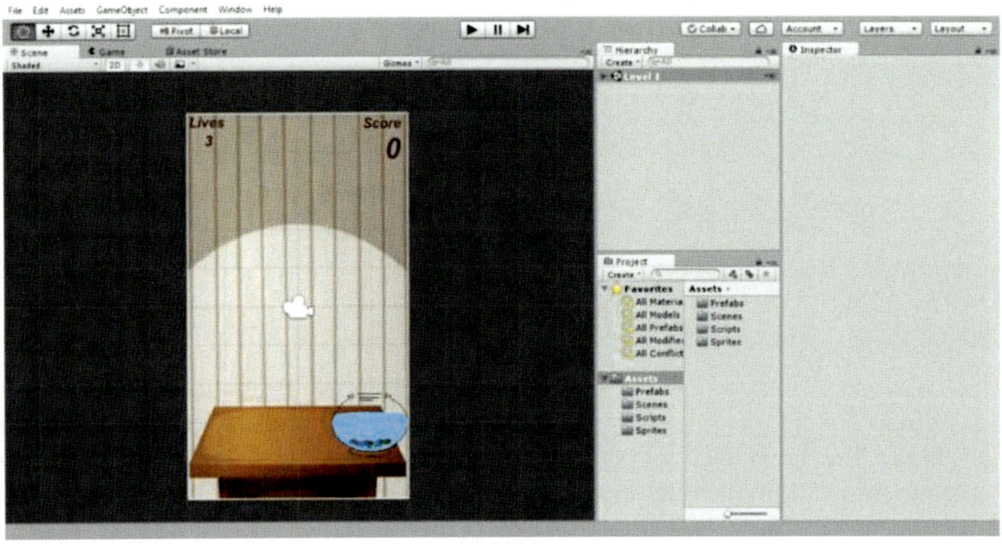

Fig. (11). Unity screen.

Methodology

Exercises Focused

The main process in rehabilitation of Hemiparesis patients include performing of therapeutic exercises. These therapeutic exercises include various exercises like

Leg exercise, Core exercise, Arm & Shoulder exercise and Hand exercise. This project mainly concentrates on Hand exercise. These hand exercises for Hemiparesis patients will support them to fine-tune their motor skills. These exercises suit well if the patient is starting with little hand movements. Until the patient can start performing on their own, these exercises can be practiced by a non-affected hand to assist the affected hand. The following stroke exercises for hands are organized from easiest Level 1 to hardest Level 3. It includes:

Level 1 (Easy)

a. Palm up and down

b. Wrist side movement

c. Rolling movement

Level 2 (medium)

d. Wrist curl movement

e. Wrist bend movement

f. Grip and release movement

Level 3 (Hard)

g. Pen spin

h. Coin drop

i. Finger curl

The physiotherapeutic exercises to augment motor activity of hemiparesis patients as shown in Fig. (**12**) and are described as follows:

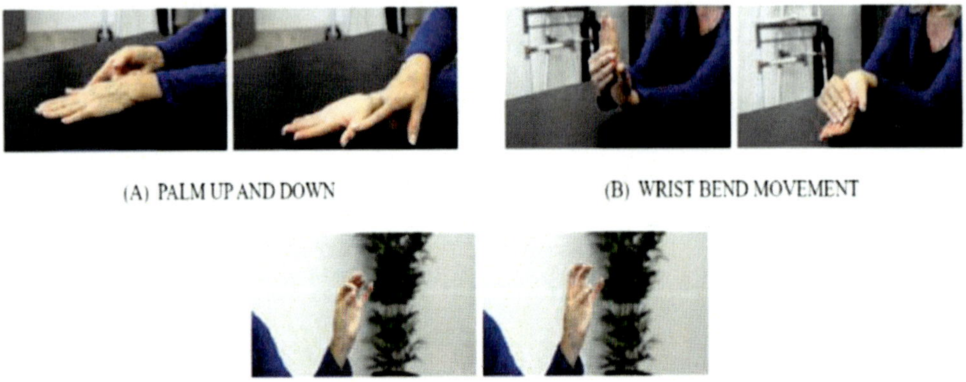

Fig. (12). Hand exercises of hemiparesis patients.

a. Palm Up and Down: The patient must place his/her hand on the top of the table with palm facing up. Next, using the unaffected hand, palm of the affected hand must be flipped down. It should be repeated back and forth. This must be repeated 10 times total.

b. Wrist Bend Movement: While keeping the patient's affected arm's elbow on the table, he/she has to use his/her unaffected hand to stretch the wrist of the affected hand. This movement should be slowly done for a whole of 5 repetitions.

c. Finger Curl: The patient must place the elbow and the affected arm on the table. He/she must perform small "O's" using fingers by taking the tip of the index finger to the tip of the thumb. The same should be repeated with the middle, ring, and pinkie finger. This must be done on all the 4 fingers for a total of 7 sets.

Games Designed

The games to augment motor activity of hemiparesis patients are designed using Unity game engine. Each game was designed based on the flexibility of the sensor usage and the ambience that promotes the rejuvenation of nerve cells (like aquarium, stars and green pastures). It includes games called fish saver (easy), blackhole mystery (medium) and whack-a-mole (hard). The games designed are shown in Fig. (**13**).

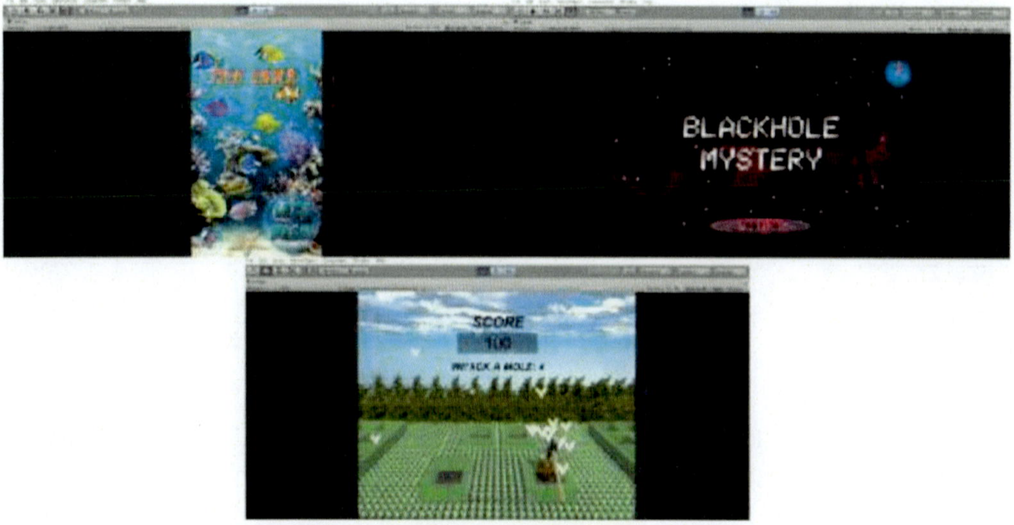

Fig. (13). Games designed for hemiparesis patients (Screenshots).

Fish Saver

This game mainly focuses on the patient to perform palm up and down exercise. It is an easy game as it only involves less motion and stamina to play. The player must move the bowl in right and left direction by flipping their palm in order to save the fishes dropping from above. Ten levels are designed in total and for each level upgraded a special sea organism is unlocked with an unknown fact. The special sea organism unlocked during each upgrade process is shown in Table **5**. These unknown facts can be asked during monthly check-up to evaluate the patient memory status.

Table 4. Arduino command symbols.

Symbol	Command	Description
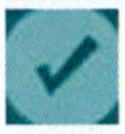	Verify	Checks code for errors compiling it.
	Upload	Compiles code and uploads it to the configured board.
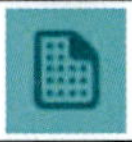	New	Creates a new sketch.
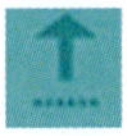	Open	Presents a menu of all the sketches in sketchbook. Clicking one will open it within the current window overwriting its content.
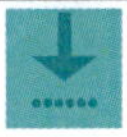	Save	Saves sketch.

(Table 4) cont.....

Symbol	Command	Description
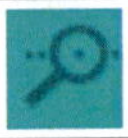	Serial Monitor	Opens the serial monitor.

Table 5. Rewards list in fish saver.

Level	Reward
1	NIL
2	Star Fish
3	Sea Horse
4	Lobster
5	Oyster
6	Crab
7	Sea Urchin
8	Stingray
9	Octopus
10	Sea Turtle

The front panel, level menu and the introduction slides of each level is shown in Fig. (**14**).

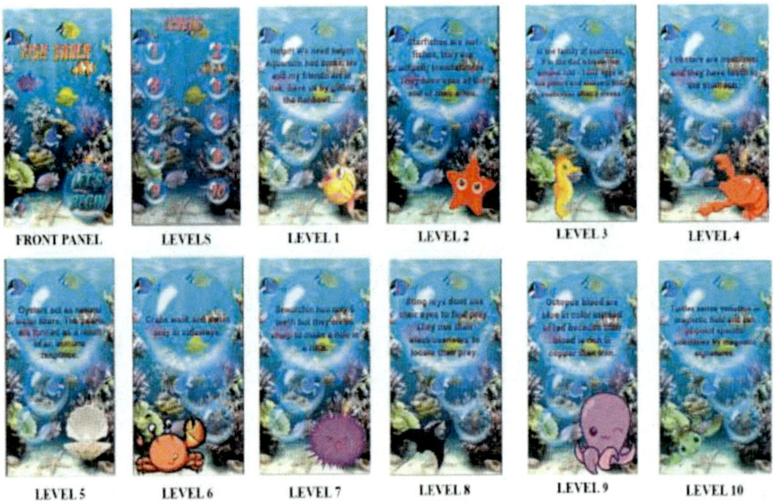

Fig. (14). Fish saver (Screenshots).

Black Hole Mystery

This game is focused for the patient to perform wrist bend movement exercise. It is a medium level game as it only involves moderate motion and stamina to play.

The player must move the blackhole in upward and downward direction by bending the wrist in order to collect the stars. Ten levels are designed in total and for each level upgraded the mystery of blackhole formation from its initial stage will be revealed. The life cycle phase or stage unlocked during each up grade process is shown in Table **6**. It also includes some unknown facts can be asked to evaluate the patient memory skill.

The different stages of stars are shown below in the Fig. (**15**),

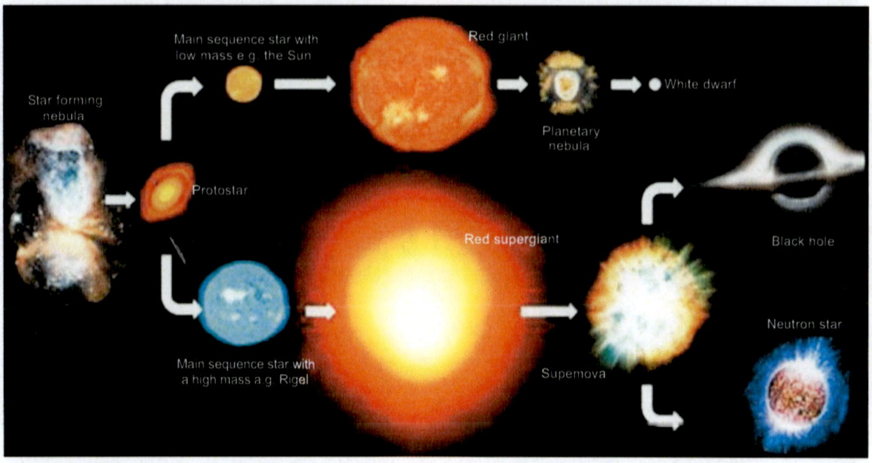

Fig. (15). Stages of star.

Table 6. Rewards list in Blackhole Mystery.

Level	Stage
1	NIL
2	Stellar Nebula
3	Protostar
4	Red Giant
5	Planetary Nebula
6	White Dwarf
7	Super Giant
8	Super Nova
9	Neutron Star
10	Blackhole

The front panel, level menu and the introduction slides of each level of blackhole mystery is shown in Fig. (**16**).

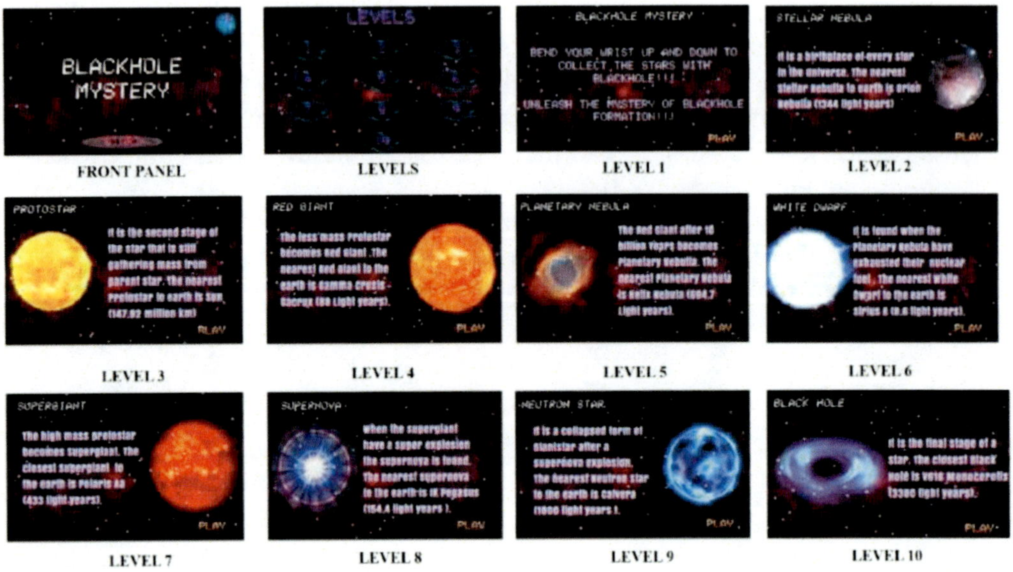

Fig. (16). Blackhole mystery (Screenshots).

Whack – A –Mole

This game is focused for the patient to perform finger curl exercise. It is a hard level game as it involves high degree of motion and more stamina to play. Once the game begin, the moles starts to pop up from their respective holes in a random fashion. The objective of this game is to push the individual moles back into their holes by hitting them directly on the head with the mallet while performing finger curl exercise. The more quickly the level is accomplished the higher the final score will be. The upgraded levels are adjusted with increase in speed thus enabling the patient to do exercise with increased motor activity. The screenshot of the designed game whack-a-mole is given in Fig. (**17**).

Block Diagram

Game Based Rehabilitation Technology

To achieve successful rehabilitation the eminent is repeating the exercises, but repeating the same movements hundreds of times does not seem exciting. Playing games let patients to make repeated, determined movements. Sometimes with constraint-induced movement and other rehabilitative methods, the patients are highly involved without being aware that they are even exercising. More participation of the patient results in increased brain activity and encourages muscle growth with increase in motor activity. Patients can play and perform these exercises using partial function or unfunctional hand with the help of functional hand every day without getting bored. At the same time, they can receive feedback about their muscle recruitment. Stroke rehabilitation also offers the opportunity for powerful knowledge translation, because the differences that was observed between stroke survivors in response to specific therapies may, in large part, be directly attribu table to differences in the brain networks supporting the desired behaviour. For the advancement of the field a knowledge of translational science is much required for the stroke rehabilitation practitioner [14-19]. Patients who are more excited about their autonomy perhaps when playing a video game are more likely to play often, work harder, and take fewer breaks than they would while doing traditional stroke recovery treatments. Affordable options are out there as already existing video game console sand touch-screen tablet sav ailable to the public. Some patients may have these existing consoles in their homes. Although it is a wonderful solution, lack of funds and difficulty in access to rehabilitative facilities and transportation often prevent patients from receiving therapy on a regular basis. The privacy and comfort of being able to receive treatment.

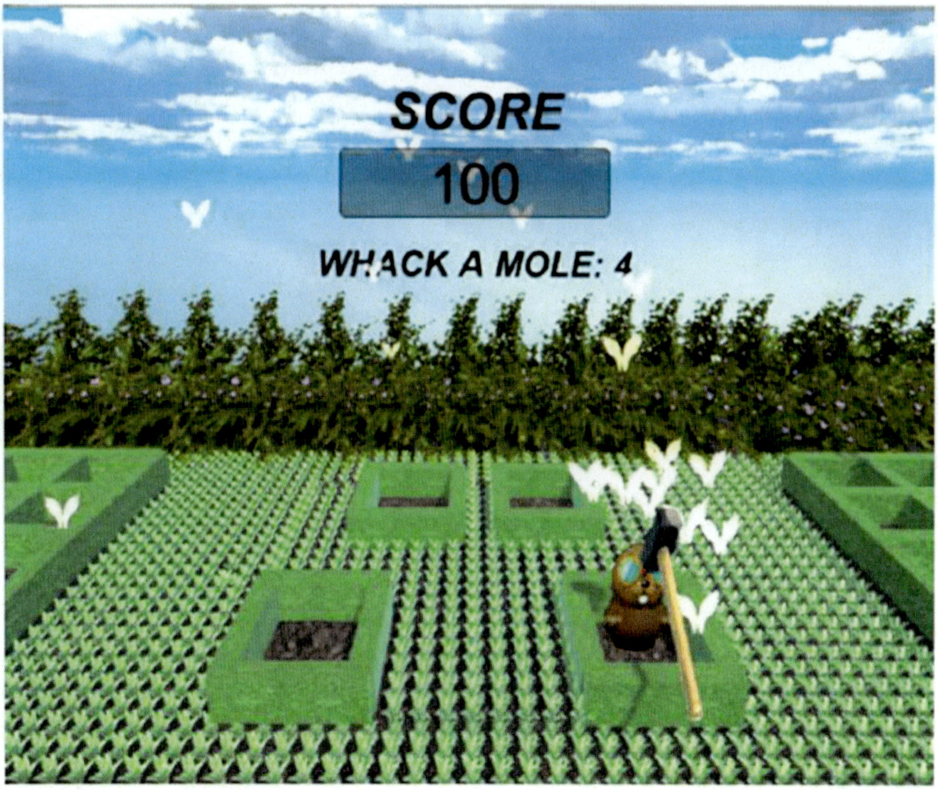

Fig. (17). Whack-a-mole (Screeenshot).

Home is the most important thing than any other, as continuation of therapy after initial, intensive rehabilitation ends and at-home participation tends to wane. Patients might choose to invite friends and family members to play with them or to watch them while playing, providing further motivation and encouragement.

There are various number of physiotherapeutic exercises available for the stroke recovery process. Of which, the developed neurorehabilitation technology aims at the neurofeedback-based gaming module to motivate the patient to perform hand exercises [20] such as palm up and down, wrist bend movement and finger curl to improve motor activities of the hand.

Developed Neurorehabilitation Technology

The developed neurorehabilitation technology employs neurorehabilitation process as an aid to improve the ADL of stroke patient. The Neuro rehabilitation is given by means of visual feedback, auditory feed back and scoring mechanism as an output of participation level of patient in doing hand exercises. The main block diagram is depicted in Fig. (**18**). The developed neuro rehabilitation technology aim store cruit the motor activities of hand in hemiparesis patients. It involves the design of type 1 glove with accelero meter and type 2g love with copperel ectrodes. The individual block diagram of components placed in respective gloves along with the microcontroller and system are shown in Figs. (**19** and **20**) respectively.

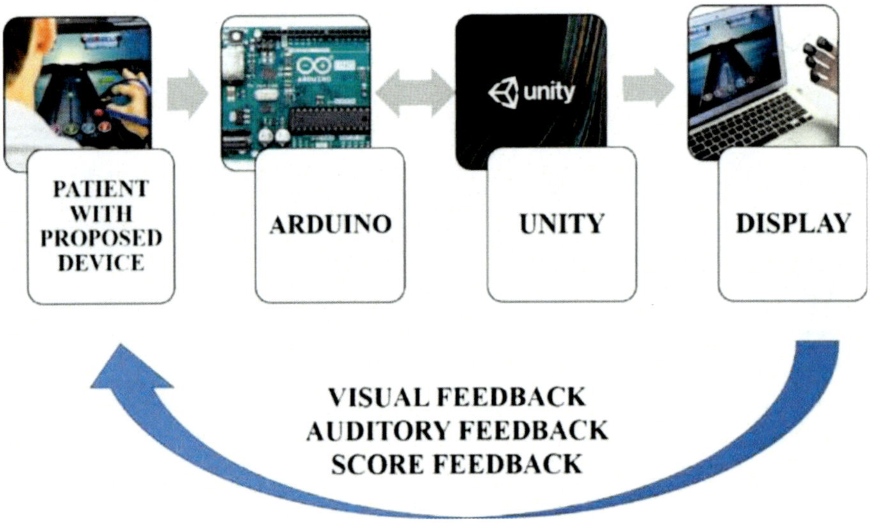

Fig. (18). Process of neurorehabilitation.

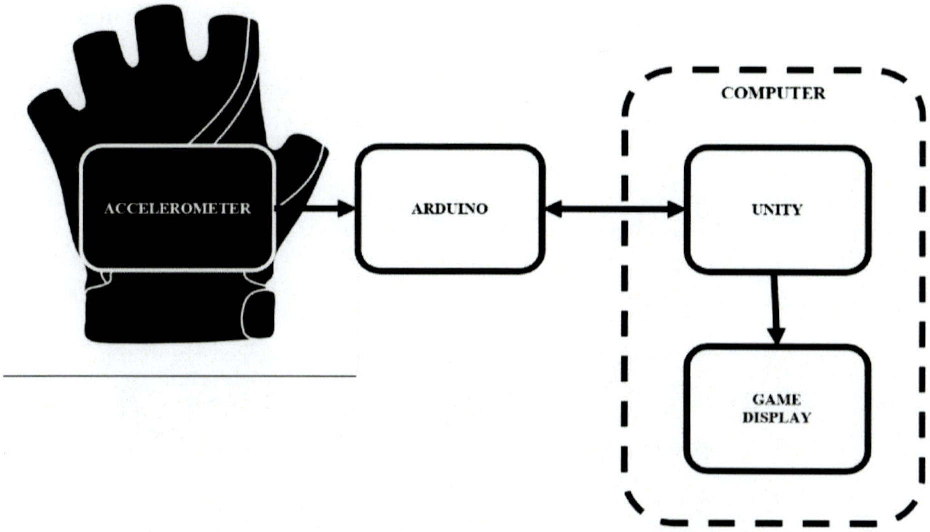

Fig. (19). Type 1 glove model.

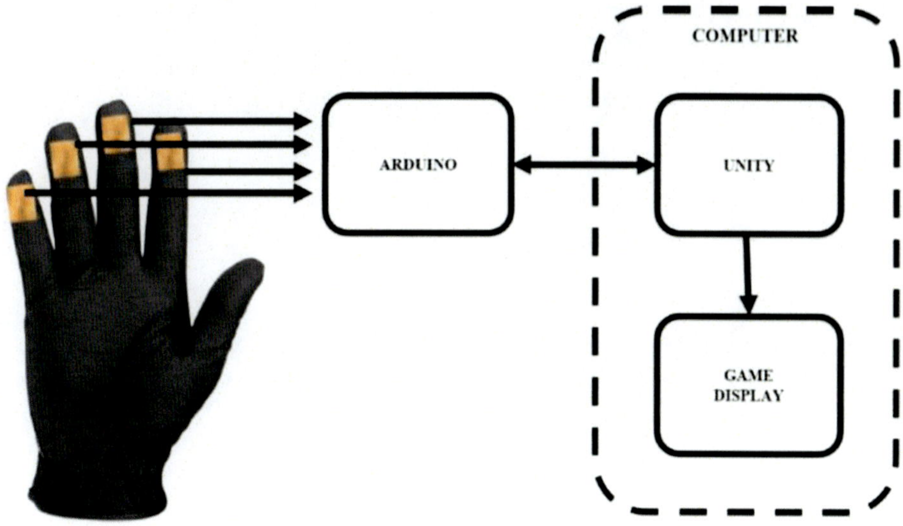

Fig. (20). Type 2 glove model.

The MEMS accelerometer sensor is connected to the patient to obtain data from the patient as he/she does palm up and down and wrist bend movement exercises. The sensor senses the translational and axial movement of limb and feeds the output to Arduino. The data obtained from Arduino is then fed to a real time engine to play games. According to the exercise performed by the patient, sensor output changes which is in turn control the interactive games displayed on a computer screen. This interactive display in turn gives visual feedback to the patient, thereby the patients can be excited to increase their game score to stepping onto the next gaming levels which indirectly increase the motor activity and full muscle recruitment that would help them in stroke recovery of hemiparesis patients. In the similar way the copper electrodes while doing finger curl exercise the capacitive sensor method toggles a microcontroller send pin to a new state and then waits for the receive pin to change to the same state as the send pin thereby giving visual feedback to the patient. The kit designed is shown in the Figs. (**21** and **22**), respectively.

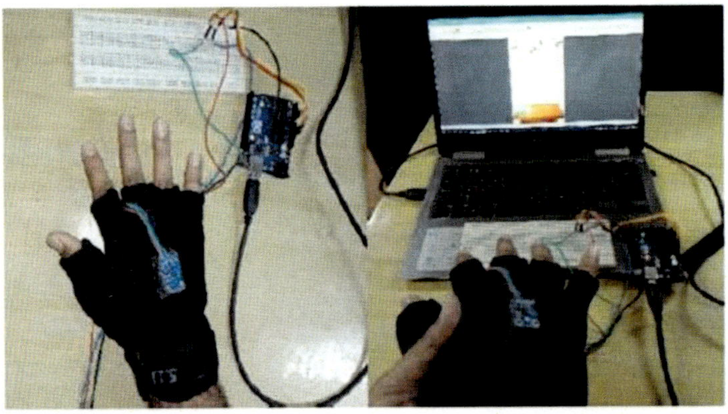

Fig. (21). Type 1 glove model kit setup.

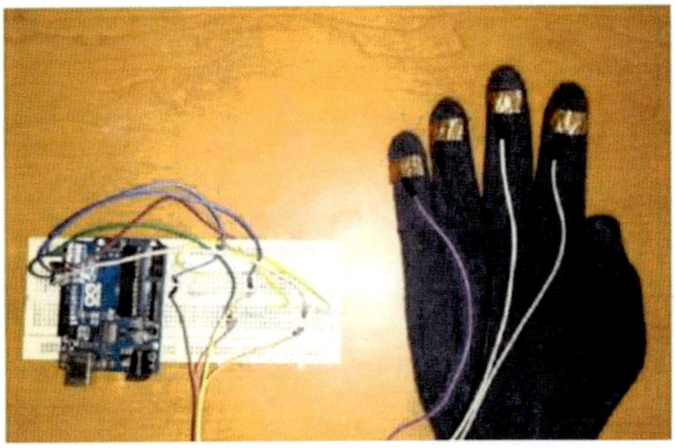

Fig. (22). Type 2 glove model kit.

Feedback

The feedbacks include visual feedback and auditory feedback. Each category is explained in the upcoming sections.

Visual Feedbacks

Visual feedback includes the change in screen when a stage or phase is achieved. For example, in the Fish Saver game when the fish is saved the water is splashed from the bowl. Also, in Blackhole Mystery when the blackhole consumes the stars few sparkles come out from its centre. In the similar way in Whack-A-Mole when the mole is hit with hammer the wings fly around. These effects are not only for designing purpose, it sometimes stimulates the player to play more and also it provides confirmation of their achievement. Each of the scene of these games are designed in order to increase the player (Hemiparesis patient) time of playing and involvement. The visual feed backs appearing in the different games are shown in Fig. (**23**).

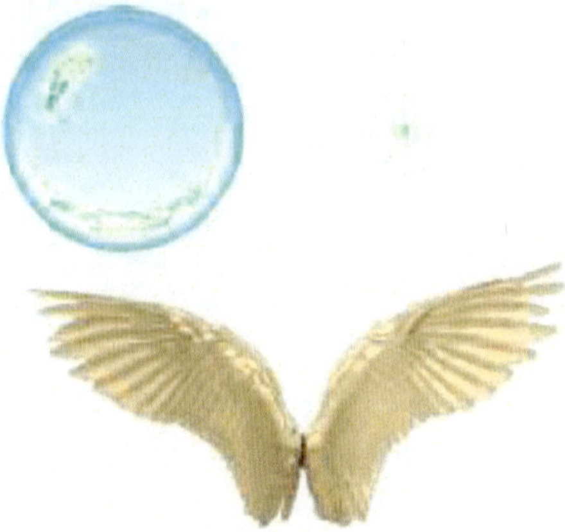

Fig. (23). Visual feedbacks (Courtesy: Wiki).

Auditory Feedback

Auditory feedback is the introduction of light to continuous music when a stage or phase is achieved. Generally, for all the games sound track are added during the introduction, level selection and level completion. In the Fish Saver game when the fish is saved the water splash music is played. There are sperate sound tracks for regular fishes and reward fishes. Also, in Blackhole Mystery when the blackhole consumes the stars bursting sound is played. It also includes sound track for regular stars and special stars unlocked at each level during the unleash of blackhole mystery. In Whack- A-Mole when the mole is hit with hammer whistle sound is played. These effects are not only for designing purpose, it also stimulates the player to play more and also it provides confirmation of their achievement. The sound tracks are added to these games so as to increase the player (Hemiparesis patient) time of playing and involvement. The audio tracks are also added at the beginning, when an option is clicked and during the level upgrade.

Score System

Score feedback is usually the process of updating the score to be viewed by the player. In the Fish Saver game when a normal fish is saved the score is added for 1 point and when a special sea organism is saved the point is updated as 2 points. In the similar way, in Blackhole Mystery when a normal star is consumed the score is added for 1point and when a special star is consumed the point is updated as 3 points. In Whack-A-Mole when the mole is hit with hammer for every hit the score is updated as10 points. These scores stimulate the player to play more and also to beat their own highs core.

EVALUATION BEFORE NEUROREHABILITATION TRAINING

The evaluation is conducted for all the subjects initially and the completed form together with the information about the subjects are given below.

Evaluation of Subject 1

The following Table **7** shows the information about the subject 1 diagnosed with Hemiparesis:

Table 7. Information about subject 1.

Form Completed By	Subject 1
Age	57
Date of birth	22.08.1962
Form completed on	01.03.2020
Training	Neurorehabilitation
Diagnosis	Left Hemiparesis

The pre-evaluation form for hemiparesis patient sheet of Subject 1 before undergoing Neurorehabilitation training gives the information regarding the subject evaluated under three categories. This form also gives the detail about the game chosen by the subject. A sample copy of pre-evaluation form is shown in Fig. (**24**).

PRE-EVALUATION FORM FOR HEMIPARESIS PATIENTS	
Basic Data	
Date:	Age:
Name:	Sex:
Examination	
BP	L ___/___ R ___/___
Pulse Rate & Rhythm	
Respiratory Rate	
History	
Last time patient w/o symptoms	Date / Time:
Mental Status	
Level of Consciousness	☐Normal ☐Abnormal
Questions (Age, Month)	☐Normal ☐Abnormal
Commands	☐Normal ☐Abnormal
Cranial Nerves	
Facial Droop	☐Left ☐Right
Visual Fields	☐Left ☐Right
Horizontal Gaze	☐Left ☐Right
Limbs	
Motor	
Arm Drift	☐Left ☐Right
Leg Drift	☐Left ☐Right
Sensory	☐Left ☐Right
Coordination	☐Left ☐Right
Conclusion	
☐Left Hemiparetic	☐Right Hemiparetic
Games Opted	
1. Fish Saver	☐Left ☐Right
2. Blackhole Mystery	☐Left ☐Right
3. Whack-A-Mole	☐Left ☐Right
Signature	Date of Session Beginning

Fig. (24). Pre-evaluation form (Sample Copy).

Evaluation of Subject 2

The following Table **8** shows the information about the subject 2 diagnosed with hemiparesis:

Table 8. Information about subject 2.

Form Completed By	Subject 2
Age	61
Date of birth	19.06.1958
Form completed on	01.03.2020
Training	Neurorehabilitation
Diagnosis	Left Hemiparesis

Evaluation of Subject 3

The following Table **9** shows the information about the subject 3 diagnosed with Hemiparesis:

Table 9. Information about subject 3.

Form Completed By	Subject 3
Age	54
Date of birth	12.12.1965
Form completed on	01.03.2020
Training	Neurorehabilitation
Diagnosis	Left Hemiparesis

Evaluation of Subject 4

The following Table **10** shows the information about the subject 4 diagnosed with Hemiparesis:

Table 10. Information about subject 4.

Form Completed By	Subject 4
Age	56
Date of birth	15.05.1963
Form completed on	01.03.2020
Training	Neurorehabilitation

(Table 10) cont.....

Form Completed By	Subject 4
Diagnosis	Right Hemiparesis

Evaluation of Subject 5

The following Table **11** shows the information about the subject 5 diagnosed with Hemiparesis:

Table 11. Information about subject 5.

Form Completed By	Subject 5
Age	63
Date of birth	12.01.1957
Form completed on	01.03.2020
Training	Neurorehabilitation
Diagnosis	Right Hemiparesis

Neurorehabilitation Training

The subject is prepared to the neurorehabilitation sessions in the following ways:

• Subject should be well rested as Neurorehabilitation requires complete involvement.

• The subject is advised to keep calm and be relaxed for about 10 minutes prior to the neurorehabilitation session.

Neurorehabilitation To Subject 1

Subject 1 was diagnosed with left hemiparesis. The subject exhibited various symptoms of Hemiparesis. The subject had a reduced motor activity in the left hand and was unable to do certain degree of motion.

Because of all these problems neurorehabilitation treatment was given to the subject. During first two sessions of training the subject was made to feel comfortable to undergo this training. The subject opted to play the games from easy to difficult level.

From the Table **12** we infer that, in the first session of Neurorehabilitation training the subject took about minutes to complete the game. But as the treatment progressed, time of completion of the game got reduced. The improvements of the subjects are discussed under Chapter. It should be noted that the subject was given neurorehabilitation for about 10 to 15 minutes in each session. If they want to perform again it was accepted.

Table 12. Neurorehabilitation to subject 1.

Session/Level	Score	Time of Completion
	Fish Saver	
1	30	00:02:18 (138s)
2	121	00:03:52 (232s)
3	142	00:04:56 (296s)
4	152	00:03:39 (219s)
5	168	00:02:15 (135s)
	Blackhole Mystery	
1	30	00:02:32 (152s)
2	139	00:03:59 (239s)
3	145	00:05:28 (328s)
4	158	00:03:43 (223s)
5	172	00:02:34 (154s)
	Whack-A-Mole	
1	190	00:02:30 (150s)
2	180	00:02:15 (135s)
3	160	00:02:00 (120s)
4	170	00:01:45 (105s)
5	140	00:01:30 (90s)

Neurorehabilitation To Subject 2

Subject 2 was diagnosed with Left Hemiparesis. The subject exhibited various symptoms of Hemiparesis. The subject had a reduced motor activity in the left hand and was unable to do his activities of daily life (ADL). Because of all these problems neurorehabilitation treatment was given to the subject. During first two sessions of training the subject was made to feel comfortable to undergo this training. The subject opted to play the games from easy to difficult level.

From the Table **13** we infer that, in the first session of Neurorehabilitation training the subject took about minutes to complete the game. But as the treatment progressed, time of completion of the game got reduced. The improvements of the subjects are discussed under Chapter. It should be noted that the subject was given neurorehabilitation for about 10 to 15 minutes in each session. If they want to perform again it was accepted.

Table 13. Neurorehabilitation to subject 2.

Session/Level	Score	Time of Completion
	Fish Saver	
1	30	00:02:22 (142s)
2	113	00:03:59 (239s)
3	138	00:05:03 (303s)
4	148	00:04:12 (252s)
5	161	00:03:01 (181s)
	Blackhole Mystery	
1	30	00:02:43 (163s)
2	127	00:04:11 (251s)
3	148	00:05:47 (347s)
4	161	00:04:08 (248s)
5	169	00:02:56 (176s)
	Whack-A-Mole	
1	170	00:02:30 (150s)
2	150	00:02:15 (135s)
3	140	00:02:00 (120s)
4	150	00:01:45 (105s)
5	120	00:01:30 (90s)

RESULT & DISCUSSION

Three games to augment hand motor activity of Hemiparesis patients have been developed. Graphical analysis of the subjects scores and time taken to complete the game *versus* the sessions undertaken of each game are discussed further.

Fish Saver

The observations of the five subjects under study based on score taken are shown in Table **14** and the observations based on time taken are shown in Table **15** for the Fish Saver game.

Table 14. Score observation of fish saver game.

Session	Subject 1	Subject 2	Subject 3	Subject 4	Subject 5
Session 1	30	30	30	30	30
Session 2	121	113	124	104	127
Session 3	142	138	146	152	148
Session 4	152	148	153	163	161
Session 5	168	161	164	175	169

Table 15. Time observation of fish saver game.

Session	Subject 1	Subject 2	Subject 3	Subject 4	Subject 5
Session 1	138	142	164	148	163
Session 2	232	239	262	247	251
Session 3	296	303	289	317	347
Session 4	219	252	292	276	248
Session 5	135	181	268	175	176

Score Analysis

• Fig. (**25**) depicts the score obtained by different subjects in Fish Saver game during different sessions.

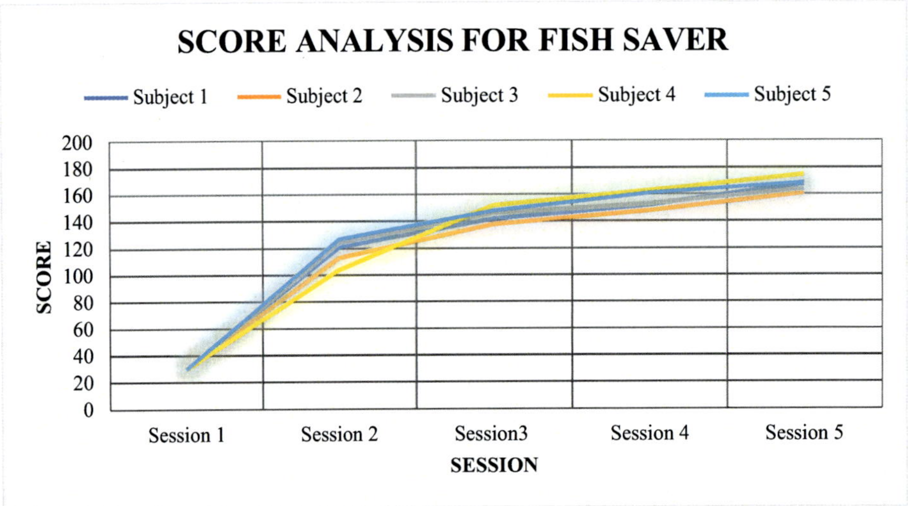

Fig. (25). Score analysis of fish saver fame.

• The scores are given for each saved fish and the rewards saved.

• There was an improvement in score obtained by them which is displayed in Y-axis and X-axis represents the sessions held.

Time Analysis

• Fig. (**26**) depicts the time taken by different subjects in Fish Saver game during different sessions.

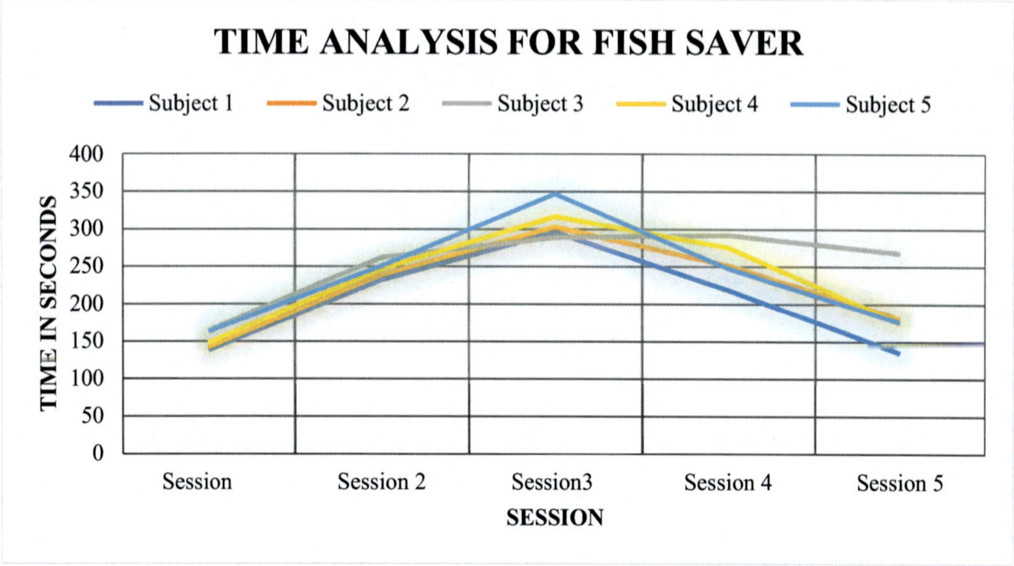

Fig. (26). Time analysis of fish saver game.

• The time was noted using stopwatch at the end of each session.

• There was a deterioration in time taken by them due to repetitive training which is displayed in Y-axis and X-axis represents the sessions held.

Blackhole Mystery

The observations of the five subjects under study based on score taken are shown in Table **16** and the observations of the five subjects based on time taken are shown in Table **17** for the Blackhole Mystery game.

Table 16. Score observation of blackhole mystery game.

Session	Subject 1	Subject 2	Subject 3	Subject 4	Subject 5
Session 1	30	30	30	30	30
Session 2	139	127	134	134	121
Session 3	145	148	153	157	142
Session 4	158	161	164	164	152
Session 5	172	169	178	175	168

Table 17. Time observation of blackhole mystery game.

Session	Subject 1	Subject 2	Subject 3	Subject 4	Subject 5
Session 1	152	163	171	182	138
Session 2	239	251	297	254	232
Session 3	328	347	309	321	296
Session 4	223	248	307	257	219
Session 5	154	176	253	164	135

Score Analysis

- The above graph (Fig. **27**) depicts the score obtained by different subjects in Blackhole Mystery game during different sessions.

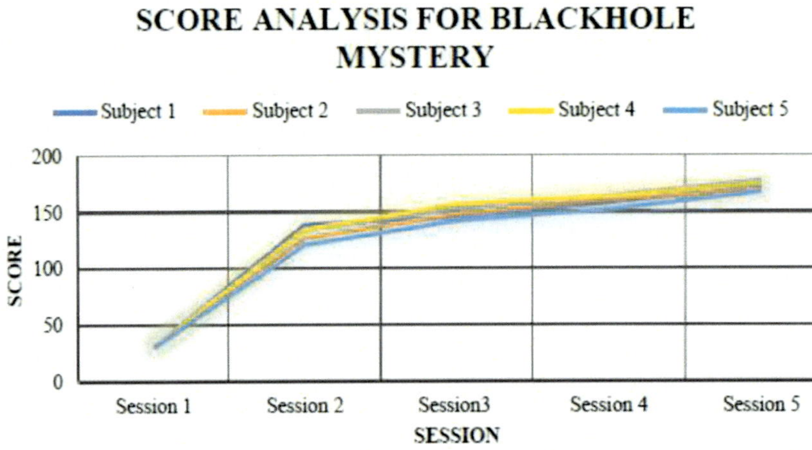

Fig. (27). Score analysis of blackhole mystery game.

• The scores are given for each star and the special stars collected.

• There was an improvement in score obtained by them which is displayed in Y-axis and X-axis represents the sessions held.

Time Analysis

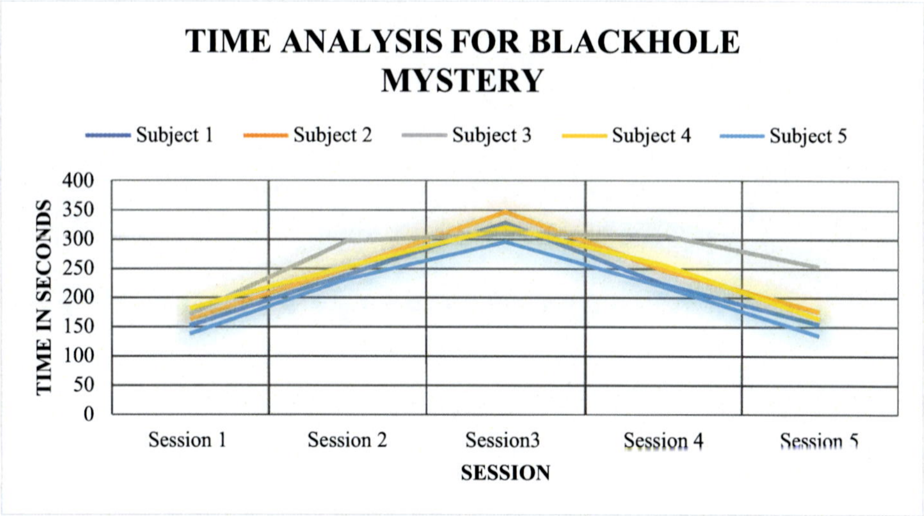

Fig. (28). Time analysis of blackhole mystery game.

• The graph in Fig. (**28**) depicts the time taken by different subjects in Blackhole Mystery game during different sessions.

• The time was noted using stopwatch at the end of each session.

• There was a deterioration in time taken by them due to repetitive training which is displayed in Y-axis and X-axis represents the sessions held.

Whack-A-Mole

The observations of the five subjects under study based on score taken are shown in Table **18** for the Whack-A-Mole game.

Table 18. Score observation of whack-a-mole game.

Session	Subject 1	Subject 2	Subject 3	Subject 4	Subject 5
Session 1	190	170	190	190	210
Session 2	180	150	140	180	160
Session 3	160	140	150	150	140
Session 4	170	150	130	160	140
Session 5	140	120	130	140	130

Score Analysis

• The graph in Fig. (**29**) depicts the score obtained by different subjects in Whack-A-Mole game during different sessions.

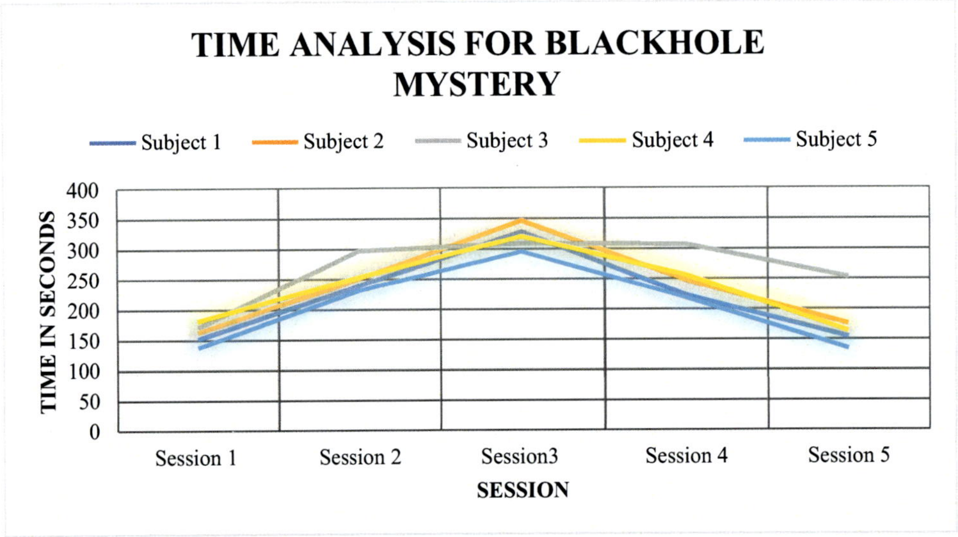

Fig. (29). Score analysis of whack-a-mole game.

• The scores are given for each hit.

• The changes in score obtained by them is displayed in Y-axis and X-axis represents the sessions held.

Through the technology developed patients are expected to continuously engage their participation in their exercise which in turn, might help them to independently perform their activities of daily life. The study observed changes in cognitive and memory and mood. The subjects showed keen interest and feedbacks are collected. It showed that there is a transition of non-functional to functional limb movement to improve the quality of activities in daily living. This project mainly aims at increasing the immersive participation of the patients. It connects patients with the games oftheir areas of interest and helps in customizing their preferred settings. While the existing rehabilitation technology tend to be much costlier, this developed neurorehabilitation gaming technology would be more cost effective and can be developed into a home based and clinic-based product.

CONCLUSION AND FUTURE WORKS

Conclusion

Worldwide, 87% of the 5.7 million deaths occur due to Stroke in low-income and middle-income countries. Hence, preventing Stroke remains a vital target in the disciplines of neurology, cardiology, vascular medicine, and geriatrics medicine. Connection of patients and customizations of games are benefits unusual of this system. High motivation increases play and exercise. In turn, improving the possibility of building new neural connections.

The greatest suggestion so far is that video games allow patients to lower their frustrations and modify the treatment protocol, which will make them more engaged. So, this proposed method would be a promising method for stroke recovery as it involves a less complicated, interactive module. Without care taker's intervention, the stroke patient would be excited as these games recall their memory of games that they played in the childhood stage as an output of cognitive improvement by rejuvenating memory cells. With this proposed interactive assistive technology, continuous participation of the patient in neurorehabilitation can lighten a few of the sequelae and assist the recovery of stroke patients. However, monotonous rehabilitation necessitates dedication to tiresome exercise routines over lengthy periods. This makes the patients leave out therapy routines. On this basis, game-based stroke rehabilitation can address two important barriers such as accessibility of rehabilitation, and patient motivation. The proposed game-based rehabilitation systems have the purpose to motivate patients to continue rehabilitation exercises at home. Further, this project showed fewer constraints, and it was cost-effective. It allows patients to select the games of their interest and customize their favored settings. It helps to continue rehabilitation exercises at home.

Future Work

- These games can be integrated with IoT (Internet of Things) to allow multiplayer mode or to have a regular update of scores online.

• Further researches can be done to design games and kits to augment motor activity other than hand including shoulder, arm, *etc*.,

CONSENT FOR PUBLICATION

Not applicable.

CONFLICT OF INTEREST

The authors declare no conflict of interest, financial or otherwise.

ACKNOWLEDGEMENT

Declared none.

REFERENCES

[1] M.E. Gurol, "Nonpharmacological management of atrial fibrillation in patients at high intracranial haemorrhage risk", *Stroke,* vol. 49, no. 1, pp. 247-254, 2018. [http://dx.doi.org/10.1161/STROKEAHA.117.017081] [PMID: 29203684]

[2] https://www.ninds.nih.gov/Disorders/Patient-Caregiver-Education/Fact-Sheets/Post-Stroke-Rehabilitation -Fact-Sheet

[3] V. Hachinski, G.A. Donnan, P.B. Gorelick, W. Hacke, S.C. Cramer, M. Kaste, M. Fisher, M. Brainin, A.M. Buchan, E.H. Lo, B.E. Skolnick, K.L. Furie, G.J. Hankey, M. Kivipelto, J. Morris, P.M. Rothwell, R.L. Sacco, S.C. Smith Jr, Y. Wang, A. Bryer, G.A. Ford, C. Iadecola, S.C.O. Martins, J. Saver, V. Skvortsova, M. Bayley, M.M. Bednar, P. Duncan, L. Enney, S. Finklestein, T.A. Jones, L. Kalra, J. Kleim, R. Nitkin, R. Teasell, C. Weiller, B. Desai, M.P. Goldberg, W.D. Heiss, O. Saarelma, L.H. Schwamm, Y. Shinohara, B. Trivedi, N. Wahlgren, L.K. Wong, A. Hakim, B. Norrving, S. Prudhomme, N.M. Bornstein, S.M. Davis, L.B. Goldstein, D. Leys, and J. Tuomilehto, "Stroke: working toward a prioritized world agenda", *Int. J. Stroke,* vol. 5, no. 4, pp. 238-256, 2010. [http://dx.doi.org/10.1111/j.1747-4949.2010.00442.x] [PMID: 20636706]

[4] FisherM, "FeuersteinG, HowellsDW, etal. Update of the stroke therapy academic industry round table preclinical recommendations", *Stroke,* vol. 40, pp. 2244-2250, 2009. [http://dx.doi.org/10.1161/STROKEAHA.108.541128] [PMID: 19246690]

[5] T.C. Hoffmann, and M.F. Walker, "'TIDieR-ing up' the reporting of interventions in stroke research: the importance of knowing what is in the 'black box'", *Int. J. Stroke,* vol. 10, no. 5, pp. 657-658, 2015. [http://dx.doi.org/10.1111/ijs.12524] [PMID: 26094670]

[6] M.F. Walker, R.J. Fisher, N. Korner-Bitensky, A. McCluskey, and L.M. Carey, WalkerMF, "FisherRJ, Korner-BitenskyN, McCluskeyA and CareyLM. From what we know to what we do: translating stroke rehabilitation research into practice", *Int. J. Stroke,* vol. 8, no. 1, pp. 11-17, 2013. [http://dx.doi.org/10.1111/j.1747-4949.2012.00974.x]

[7] S.I. Savitz, S.C. Cramer, L. Wechsler, J. Aronowski, J. Boltze, C. Borlongan, C. Case, T. Chase, M. Chopp, S.T. Carmichael, S.C. Cramer, P. Duncan, S. Finklestein, S. Fischkoff, R. Guzman, D.C. Hess, D. Huang, J. Hinson, S. Kautz, D. Kondziolka, R. Mays, V. Misra, P. Mitsias, M. Modo, K. Muir, S.I. Savitz, J. Sinden, E. Snyder, G. Steinberg, F. Vahidy, L. Wechsler, A. Willing, S. Wolf, E. Yankee, and D.R. Yavagal, STEPS 3 Consortium, "Stem cells as an emerging paradigm in stroke 3: enhancing the development of clinical trials", *Stroke,* vol. 45, no. 2, pp. 634-639, 2014. [http://dx.doi.org/10.1161/STROKEAHA.113.003379] [PMID: 24368562]

[8] M. Ali, C. English, and J. Bernhardt, "", *More outcomes than trials: a call for consistent data collection across stroke rehabilitation trials. Int J Stroke.*, vol. 8, pp. 18-24, 2013.

[9] https://insights.patientbond.com/blog/how-technology-is-changing-stroke-rehabilitation

[10] Gazihan Alankus, "Motion-based video games for stroke rehabilitation with reduced compensatory motions", *All theses and dissertations (etds).*, p. 547, 2011.

[11] N Barrett, I Swain, and C Gatzidis, "The use and effect of video game design theory in the creation of game-based systems for upper limb stroke rehabilitation", *Journal of rehabilitation and assistive technologies engineering.*, vol. 3, pp. 1-16, 2015.

[12] Y Hung, P Huang, and K Chen, "What do stroke patients look for in game-based rehabilitation", *Medicine observational study.*, vol. 95, 2016. [http://dx.doi.org/10.1097/MD.0000000000003032]

[13] B Valde, S Glegg, and N Lambertshirzad, "Application of commercial games for home-based rehabilitation for people with hemiparesis: challenges and lessons learned", *Games for health journal.* Vol 7: Chapter 3 (Mar 2018).

[14] L.J. Gonzalez Rothi, and A.M. Barrett, "Treatment innovation in behavioral rehabilitation of stroke: Removing limits on recovery", *J. Rehabil. Res. Dev.*, vol. 43, no. 3, pp. vii-x, 2006. [http://dx.doi.org/10.1682/JRRD.2006.08.0086] [PMID: 17041815]

[15] A.M. Barrett, C.E. Levy, and L.J.G. Rothi, "Treatment innovation in rehabilitation of cognitive and motor deficits after stroke and brain injury: physiological adjunctive treatments", *Am. J. Phys. Med. Rehabil.*, vol. 86, no. 6, pp. 423-425, 2007. [http://dx.doi.org/10.1097/PHM.0b013e31805ba039] [PMID: 17515680]

[16] A.M. Barrett, C.E. Levy, and L.J. Gonzalez Rothi, "Pharmaceuticals for poststroke and brain injury rehabilitation", *Am. J. Phys. Med. Rehabil.*, vol. 86, no. 8, pp. 603-604, 2007. [http://dx.doi.org/10.1097/PHM.0b013e3181148ce0] [PMID: 17667189]

[17] L.J. Gonzalez-Rothi, "Cognitive Rehabilitation", *J. Head Trauma Rehabil.*, vol. 21, no. 2, pp. 194-197, 2006. [http://dx.doi.org/10.1097/00001199-200603000-00011] [PMID: 16569992]

[18] R.P. Van Peppen, G. Kwakkel, S. Wood-Dauphinee, H.J. Hendriks, P.J. Van der Wees, and J. Dekker, "The impact of physical therapy on functional outcomes after Stroke: what's the evidence? Clin Rehabil2004;18:833–862. [19]. Kwakkel G, Kollen BJ, Lindeman E. Understanding the pattern of functional recovery after Stroke: facts and theories", *Restor. Neurol. Neurosci.*, vol. 22, pp. 281-299, 2004.

[20] Available at: https://www.flintrehab.com/product/musicglove-hand-therapy/

[21] E.L. Deci, H. Eghrari, B.C. Patrick, and D.R. Leone, "Facilitating internalization: the self-determination theory perspective", *J. Pers.*, vol. 62, no. 1, pp. 119-142, 1994. [http://dx.doi.org/10.1111/j.1467-6494.1994.tb00797.x] [PMID: 8169757]

CHAPTER 11

Smart Wearable Sensor Design Techniques For Mobile Health Care Solutions

K. Vijaya[1,*] and **B. Prathusha Laxmi**[2]

[1] *SRM Institute of Science and Technology, Chennai, India*

[2] *R.M.K. Engineering College, Chennai, India*

Abstract: In this chapter, we discuss the technological developments that have led to the clinical utility of smart wearable body sensors. Smart wearable sensors can enhance the physician-patient relationship, promote remote monitoring techniques, and their impact on healthcare management and expenditure. We explore how continuous health status monitoring can be achieved with the help of wireless sensors, wireless communication, microprocessors, and data processing algorithms. Furthermore, we also discuss the impact of using wearable sensor systems by infants and aged persons to alert parents/caretakers/clinicians. We also explore integrating smart wearable sensors and IoT to enhance the automatic monitoring and alerting systems for health care improvement.

Keywords: Alerting, Communication, Healthcare, Monitoring, Sensors, Vital parameters, Wearable, Wireless.

INTRODUCTION TO THE SENSOR TECHNOLOGY

A sensor is a device that will receive and respond to signals that could be produced by heat, light, motion, or chemical reactions. Sensors detect the presence of energy, energy changes, and energy transfer with the help of a transducer and convert the signals into readable format. Thermal sensors are used to gauge the environment's absolute temperature, how it affects two different metals, and the heat generated by chemical processes. Some mechanical sensors are meant to measure pressure, altitude, acceleration, and flow rate of liquid or gas. Electrical sensors are used for measuring resistance, voltage, current, and amount of electricity supplied/consumed. Chemical sensors are used for identifying the amount of oxygen present in the liquid or gas being analysed. Furthermore, they are used to identify the presence of carbon dioxide and any other as that needs to be monitored. Optical sensors are used to detect light,

* **Corresponding author K. Vijaya:** SRM Institute of Science and Technology, Chennai, India; Tel: 9444146212; E-mail: vijayak@srmist.edu.in

electromagnetic energy, the intensity of light, and infra-red radiation. Acoustic sensors are meant to measure seismic waves and wave velocity in the air or an environment. Apart from the above-mentioned sensors, we have motion sensors for detecting motion and sensors for measuring speed, atomic radiation, and monitoring human cells.

Biological sensors can measure carbohydrates, alcohol, acids, blood sugar levels, and air and water quality. They can also detect pathogens. Hence, they can be used for pollution control, general health monitoring, screening, analysis, and diagnosis of diseases. The materials used in biosensors [1] can be categorized into biocatalytic group (enzyme), bio-affinity group (antibodies, nucleic acid), and microbes (microorganism). Biosensors can be based on enzymes, tissues, immune systems, magnetic fields, heat, piezoelectricity, light, peptides, proteins, DNA, and genetic encoding. Biosensing technology has penetrated the food industry, agriculture, marine, defence, and clinical sector. In the medical field, biosensors are employed for a variety of purposes, including drug discovery, the diagnosis of viral and metabolic illnesses, the early detection of human interleukin, and the probing of gene expression. Nanomaterial-based biosensors [2] have outstanding physical and chemical properties and are being used for drug delivery [3], cancer treatment [4], and catalysis [5].

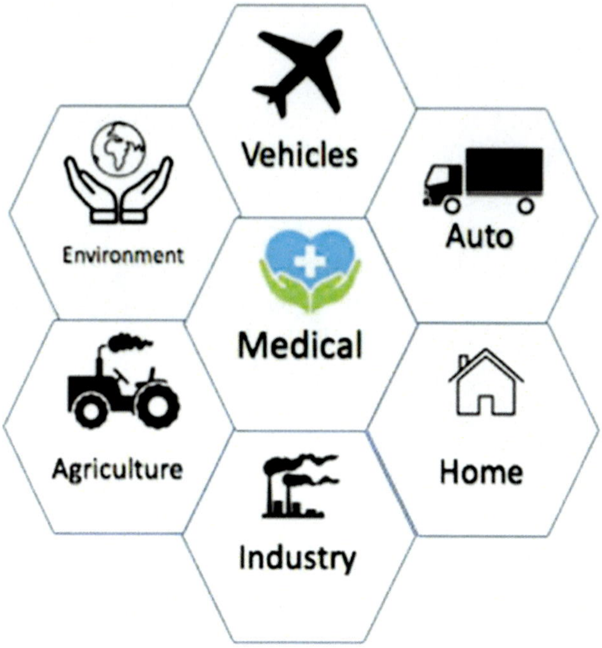

Fig. (1). Application of sensors.

Sensor technology has led to the development of devices that are used to acquire information based on the physical, chemical, or biological properties of an object and convert it into readable signals. Sensors are prominently used for measuring temperature, colour, gas, light, smoke, humidity, touch, soil moisture, IR, Ultrasonic, water flow, rain, heartbeat, proximity, EEG, conductance, and inertial. Sensors are ubiquitous and are at homes, offices, cars, and other work and living places to enhance our standard of living. Some of the common applications of sensors are turning on/off lights, room temperature adjustment, smoke or fire detection, garage door opening, and coffee making, as shown in Fig. (**1**).

DIFFERENT TYPES OF SENSORS AND THE PHYSIOLOGICAL PARAMETERS THEY COULD DETECT

Depending on the placement of sensors, they could be categorised as environmental, wearable, and implanted, as shown in Fig. (**2**). Moreover, Fig. (**3**) shows different types of sensors. Environmental sensors are generally used for measuring air temperature, humidity, air quality, pressure, dust concentration, light, and noise. Air monitoring of the environment will help us identify the level of contaminants to which a patient undergoing surgery will be exposed. Temperature sensors are used to adjust the working of the electronic gadgets to ensure that appropriate temperature is maintained so that the food in the warehouse, drugs in pharmaceutical storage, and their transportation are maintained appropriately. Humidity sensors are used in office environments for heating, ventilating, and cooling system control, generally used along with temperature sensors. Light sensors are used to automatically illuminate the rooms and control the intensity of the light. Motion sensors enable us to detect unauthorized movement in restricted areas and open doors automatically for thoroughfare entries.

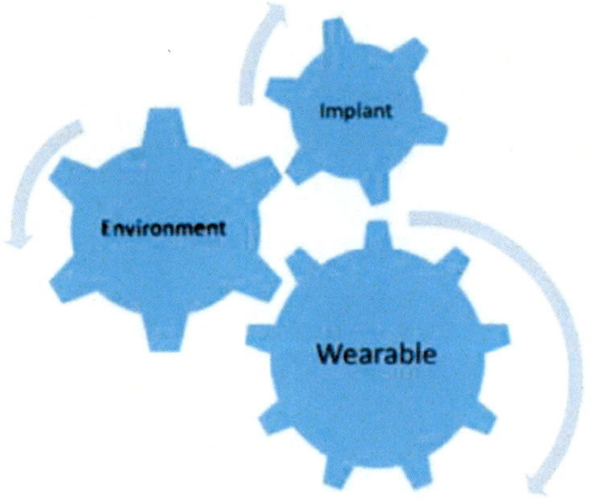

Fig. (2). Placement of sensors.

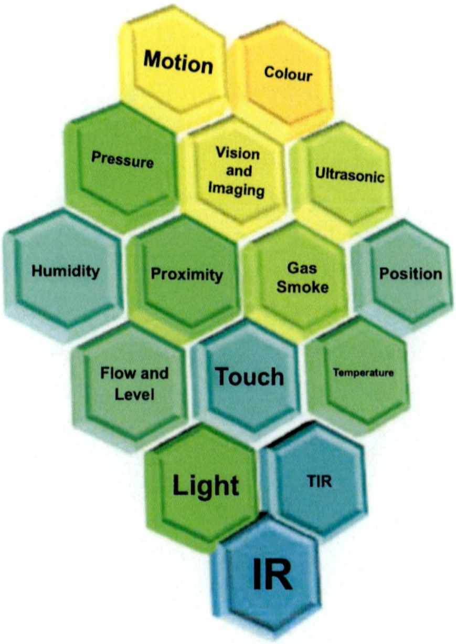

Fig. (3). Types of sensors.

Environmental sensors are connected objects that could be used for measuring air quality. Due to their static positioning, the data received from sensors at the monitoring stations might not be accurate enough compared to the data collected through environmental sensors. Having specific real-time information will help in identifying the reason for pollution in a specific area so that a proper mitigation plan could be devised to alleviate pollution. Some of the portable environmental sensor devices that have been developed in the recent past are airbot, waterbot, sensordrone, lapka, sensaris, air quality egg, electronic nose, pressurenet, and broadcom microchip [6].

Implantable sensors [7] and devices, like pacemakers, cardioverter defibrillators, and deep brain simulators, have been used as treatment options for patients. The pacemaker monitors heartbeat, and if the moment irregularity is identified, it provides low-energy electrical pulses to restore the rate of heartbeat. The cardioverter-defibrillator is an advanced version of a pacemaker that provides high-energy electrical pulses if it is not possible to restore the rhythm of the heartbeat by providing low-energy electrical pulses. Deep brain simulators are used to provide electrical signals that control movement for patients with Parkinson's disease. Battery-less, biodegradable, organic photodetectors, organic light-emitting diode, micro light-emitting diode, and electrocorticography electrodes are some of the advancements in implantable sensors.

Wearable sensors have opened up a new dimension of health care administration and enhanced the lifestyle of humans. Integration of wearable sensors and mobile technology has revolutionised the way doctors and patients contribute to the health care of individuals. Though remotely monitoring a patient has been in use for quite some time, the invention of smart wearable body sensors has taken this to the next level. For more than a decade, researchers have started working on integrating different sensors to design and develop wearable devices that could reduce the human effort required for continuous monitoring of patients, both in-house and remote mode. Many researchers are working in this domain as the devices available for consumers are increasing tremendously. The evidence for reliability of these devices is increasingly available and can be accessed.

Heart rate could be used to identify the risk of coronary artery disease, stroke, sudden death, and non-cardiovascular diseases [8]. ECG sensors could be used to detect various heart problems [9]. The prevalence of health problems in India is due to unhealthy lifestyles, increasing levels of stress and pollution, and a low doctor-patient ratio. The health care sector is one of the fastest-growing sectors in the world. However, accessibility and cost are the major limiting factors to address health issues. It is indicated that only around 19% of the Indian urban population have health insurance coverage, and around 9% of urban India develop major health problems.

According to the literature, telemedicine is being adopted to care for patients with cardiac diseases, diabetes, hypo and hypertension, and hypo and hyperthermia [10]. Sensors can be used for monitoring chronic illnesses, like asthma, heart failure, cardiopulmonary disease, as they need continuous long-term monitoring to avoid the threat to life. Extensive research has been carried out to study the utilization of smartphones for continuous monitoring, sharing, and maintaining health records and also inbuilt apps that could be used [11 - 16] for health care monitoring remotely. There is an increase in the usage of remote monitoring systems, indicating an increase in the data volume. Hence, it would be possible to accelerate the patient rehabilitation process and promote a better diagnosis of diseases.

For more accurate, reliable, cost-effective wearable devices, biosensors can be used. Cardiac patients can be monitored continuously using Wireless Sensor Networks. By monitoring remotely using wireless sensor wearable devices, various goals can be achieved, such as avoiding long stays at the hospital and decreasing costs. The working of a wireless sensor device in a wearable smart device depends on the wireless sensor nodes attached to the patient's body for sensing vital parameters. The data collected through the sensors are processed and communicated to the control unit, where data is stored, processed, and displayed.

When there is a need to communicate the data for longer distances, appropriate internet devices need to be used.

INTRODUCTION TO WIRELESS SENSORS COMMUNICATION

Diseases, like cardiovascular and cerebrovascular, need continuous monitoring of few parameters, requiring a stay at the hospital for a long duration. Hospital staff monitors patient's condition continuously using medical devices like wired monitors. These wired monitors are uncomfortable to patients as they need to stay at the hospital for a long duration, and a high cost is involved during their stay. Nowadays, the health monitoring system uses wearable devices consisting of sensors that monitor different parameters, such as temperature, respiratory rate, heart rate, *etc*.

Many researchers have come up with the idea of wearables to monitor various vital parameters, like heart rate, cardiac activity during sleep, and chronic wound monitoring. For example, researchers have proposed a heart attack detection system using ZigBee devices to monitor heart-related parameters. Using mobile devices, like smartphones, we can detect, store, and perform analysis of collected records.

Smart step is a footwear-based wearable device that is used for activity monitoring with the help of smart phone. 6LowPAN is a protocol that could be used to communicate the vital sign data collected through body area network onto the Internet. ESP8266 wi-fi module could be used to communicate the data to another ESP8266 wi-fi module without using Internet.

INTEGRATION OF SENSORS AND OTHER RELATED TECHNOLOGIES TO CREATE SMART WEARABLE DEVICE

To create smart wearable devices using sensors, many components need to be integrated with many state-of-the-art technologies. These technologies need a collaboration of various disciplines, like material science, electrical engineering, and mechanical engineering. Wearable materials are to be decided based on the type and purpose of the device; material scientists need to work on the type of material that should be used to fabricate the sensor. For the devices to be working properly, a power supply is essential; therefore, there is a need to decide the right type of battery used for a specific device by an electrical engineer. The size of the battery should be minimal, and the battery life should be long. Recently, several research works have been carried out on sustainable battery technology. A battery-free, wireless optoelectronic system has been reported earlier [17]; in this work, near-field communication technology and magnetic inductive coupling were used to power up the device.

Antenna technology is used to communicate the sensor data to a communication module as most of the wearable devices are meant to be used for remote monitoring. This communication module can be an integration of gateways involving the internet or a telecommunication system. Wireless communication technology plays a vital role in transporting the sense data from the wearable device to the central server. The tremendous number of improvements in antenna and wireless technology have made the use of remote monitoring wearables a trending and successful healthcare system model.

Technologies, like Bluetooth, ZigBee, and near-field communication and remarkable improvements in the design of flexible devices have made it possible to access remote health care through mobile devices. Advancements in mobile technology have also contributed to the advancements in remote health care systems. Bluetooth technology has gained attention in the field of wireless wearable sensors due to its low cost. Moreover, it consumes less power, and the line-of-sight issue is not there. Extensive research has been carried out, and miniaturization of Bluetooth modules and improvement of mutual transfer performance have led to designing wearable devices with integrated Bluetooth modules.

Integration of embedded systems, wireless sensor networks, control systems automation, and convergence of technologies, like analytics, machine learning, and sensors have made IoT technology a major contributor to the recent developments in medical care. Internet of Medical Things, also referred to as smart healthcare, is the technology used to create a digitized health care system that can be used to connect medical resources and healthcare services. Extensive research is being carried out by researchers across the world to devise smart healthcare systems that can be used by medical practitioners to provide proactive treatment for patients.

DIFFERENT WEARABLE DEVICES THAT HAVE BEEN DESIGNED AND USED

Infants and Adults

Specifically, it is essential for us to have health care monitoring systems that address the issues of monitoring infants and elders. Infants are not able to communicate their state; hence sensors would be helpful in identifying their vital parametric values. As far as elders are concerned, they usually do not communicate about the change in their vital parameters, as they do not want their loved ones to panic. Oftentimes, it is too late by the time they discuss their condition.

Continuous monitoring of the infants is essential for detecting and preventing many diseases, as they cannot express their pain and uneasiness. Hence, it is very important to continuously monitor their vital signs when they are born prematurely or critically ill to avoid extreme outcomes. Recent advancements in wearable technology have led to the development of systems for monitoring the health condition of infants. More than twenty-two state-of-the-art wireless infant health monitoring systems have been developed. Furthermore, a smart neonatal jacket can be used to monitor the ECG reading of infants and display the outcome on laptops.

Fig. (**4**) represents one of the architectures that can be used to implement a health monitoring system for an infant. Depending on the purpose of monitoring, the parameters to be monitored should be decided, and biosensors should be placed in one of the many wearable devices that can be used on infants. The data gathered using the sensor should be communicated using appropriate networking devices to the processing unit. The processing unit performs computations based on the parametric values received from the biosensors [18], communicates, and stores them in the database. The processing unit also identifies whether a notification or an alert needs to be sent. Depending on the processed data, it will either send an alert message or notification to the parent and doctor. An alert message will be sent as an MMS to the registered mobile and mail IDs of parents and doctors.

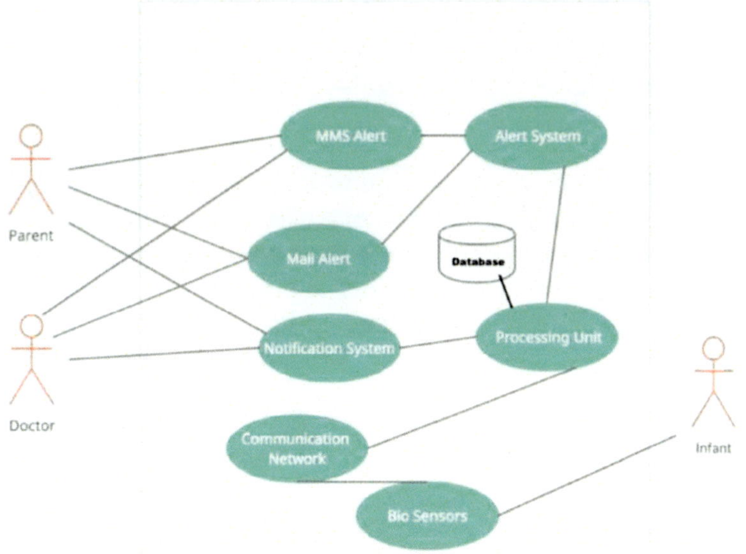

Fig. (4). Architecture of health monitoring system for infant.

To facilitate working parents to monitor their infants, there is a wearable pair of socks to continuously monitor the temperature and heartbeat of the infants. The system remotely captures the information and sends it to a mobile application. Parents can install that application and get alerts and notifications in case of an emergency. This wearable system gives an edge over traditional health monitoring approaches. This approach reduces the human workforce and also helps in capturing several vital parameters necessary for decision-making. Table **1** shows multiple parameters that can be monitored using wearable devices in health care for infants.

Table 1. Parameters to be monitored in infants using wearable devices.

Parameter	Description	Health Condition
ECG	Measurement of the electrical activity in an infant's heart	Cardiovascular Disease
Heart rate	Measurement of heartbeats per minute	Tachycardia, bradycardia
Respiratory rate	Measurement of the number of breaths per minute	Apnea, hypopnea, tachypnea
Body temperature	Measurement of temperature	Hypothermia, hyperthermia
Hydration	Measurement of water levels	Diarrhoea, vomiting
Body movements	Detection of motion	Range of motion, SIDS

Wearable Infant Health Monitoring System can be used for single-parameter health monitoring or multiple-parameter health monitoring. Single-parameter health monitoring systems are meant for monitoring specific parameters, like ECG, heart rate, respiratory rate, and other relevant parameters.

Heart Rate Monitoring: It is an important parameter for identifying heart-related issues in infants. It is very critical to monitor the heart rate [19] of the infant to detect heartbeat-related issues, such as tachycardia and bradycardia. RFID-based technology wearable device is used to monitor the heart rate of infants, and information captured is sent to the android application for display. Additionally, in this system, an alarm system is connected locally with the processing unit to notify when there is a loss of signal or the range (80 – 180 bpm) deviates.

Respiratory Monitoring: It is defined as the number of breaths taken per minute. It is very difficult to monitor this parameter. There are many wearable devices to monitor the number of breaths taken by infants and identify a reduction of breath or abnormally fast breathing. One of such devices is an RFID-based wearable device to monitor the respiratory system of the infant. It is designed in a way that it is wrapped around the belly for detecting motion-based artifacts. In this device, movements of the chest wall and abdomen are used for measuring the breathing rate.

In multiple parameter health monitoring, the scope is broadened so that the device can monitor multiple health parameters of the infants. For example, a smart jacket is able to monitor the vital signs of infants. The smart jacket is embedded with different textile sensors to monitor multiple parameters. Another example is a chest belt used to monitor infants continuously in their sleep to detect SIDS.

Smart health care monitoring system [20] involves multiple users, *viz.* doctors, patients, hospitals, and research organizations. It is a system with multiple advantages, like monitoring, preventing, and diagnosing diseases, providing treatment, managing hospital systems, decision-making in health-related scenarios. It has applications in the field of medical research and information technology. Some of the technologies that play a major role in the smart health care system include the Internet of Things, Wireless communication, Cloud computing, Artificial Intelligence. From patient's perspective, they can use a variety of wearable devices [21] to continuously monitor their health and take necessary steps, if required, through virtual assistants. From the doctor's perspective, these devices will help them monitor their patients from anywhere and perform diagnoses to administer treatment. Doctors can maintain medical records of the patient in an integrated platform for continuous monitoring, irrespective of where they are.

During extreme climatic conditions, there is a possibility that elders are prone to get affected by dehydration, lung infection and antibiotic-resistant infections. With the advent of sensors for monitoring many of the health parameters like temperature, skin conductance, electrocardiograms, electromyograms, electroencephalograms, identifying infectious people during the pandemic was made possible. If sensors are used to monitor the heart rate, blood pressure, blood glucose, body temperature and other physiological parameters of a person [22] it is possible to alert the physicians or well-wishers through the wireless technology.

With innovations in health care management, the world's population is increasingly aging, and it is projected that by 2050, the number of people aged above 65 years might reach 1548.9 million and above 80 might reach 109.1 million. This makes it necessary for us to come up with better healthcare management for the elderly population. The most prominent ailments that need to be handled among the aging population are dementia, Alzheimer's [23], Parkinson's, cardiovascular, and frailty. As there is a constant need to monitor and support elders with the aforementioned ailments, integration of technologies, like sensors, IoT, data analytics, and AI, is essential. A study by Wang reviewed indoor positioning systems, emphasizing human activity recognition and biometric sensors (vital sign monitoring, blood pressure, and glucose).

Fall Detection systems had been investigated by Fang-Yie [24]. Data from the accelerometer are evaluated with several threshold-based algorithms and position data to determine a fall. The threshold is adaptive based on parameters, such as height, weight, and level of activity, provided by users. Dementia [25] disease is detected by wearable IAT that can track and detect moments of significance for individuals with dementia. As dementia is associated with progressively declining cognitive and motor abilities, this IAT focuses upon detecting significant moments from their physiological signals.

Many case studies have been carried out on fall detection, fall prediction, wandering detection, symptom detection, GAIT analysis, dementia, intervention, and assessment. A wearable ring-type pulse monitoring sensor [26] can be integrated with a smartphone so that the user can monitor his/her pulse and temperature.

Parkinson's disease is a brain disorder. Wearable technology is reliable in real-time monitoring of tremor [27 - 33], frozen gait [34 - 44], movement disorder [45 - 50], and rigidity [51] in experimental and familial environments [52, 53].

Most elderly people are haunted by age-related diseases. With the help of real-time monitoring, we can monitor some of the health parameters of patients in their home environment instead of monitoring them at the hospital. Vital signs of an individual can be monitored regularly and can be altered by both individuals and health caretakers. Wearable monitoring sensors focus on biosignals, *viz.*, body temperature, heart rate, respiration rate, blood pressure, and pulse oxygenation. Wearable sensors have a better interface with human skin. Silicon-based electronic devices are used for data processing and communication for the purpose of monitoring and alarming the system. Wearable sensor together with silicon-based electronic devices consumes less power and works for long duration to support mobility. Bio-data collected from sensors are processed to predict, diagnose, and make decisions for a healthy life. Sensor-based technologies are mostly used for elderly persons that involve accelerometers and gyroscopes.

Fig. (**5**) illustrates functions that are associated with the design of wearable devices for aged people. Various technologies are associated with collecting data from physical activity, precise positioning, and vital monitoring. A software system that consists of modules for data processing, extraction of features, recognition of physical activity, and decision making must be developed. Bio-mechanical sensors monitor various health parameters integrated into a prototype of aged people, and this prototype configured with multiple sensors can be incorporated into clothing worn by aged persons.

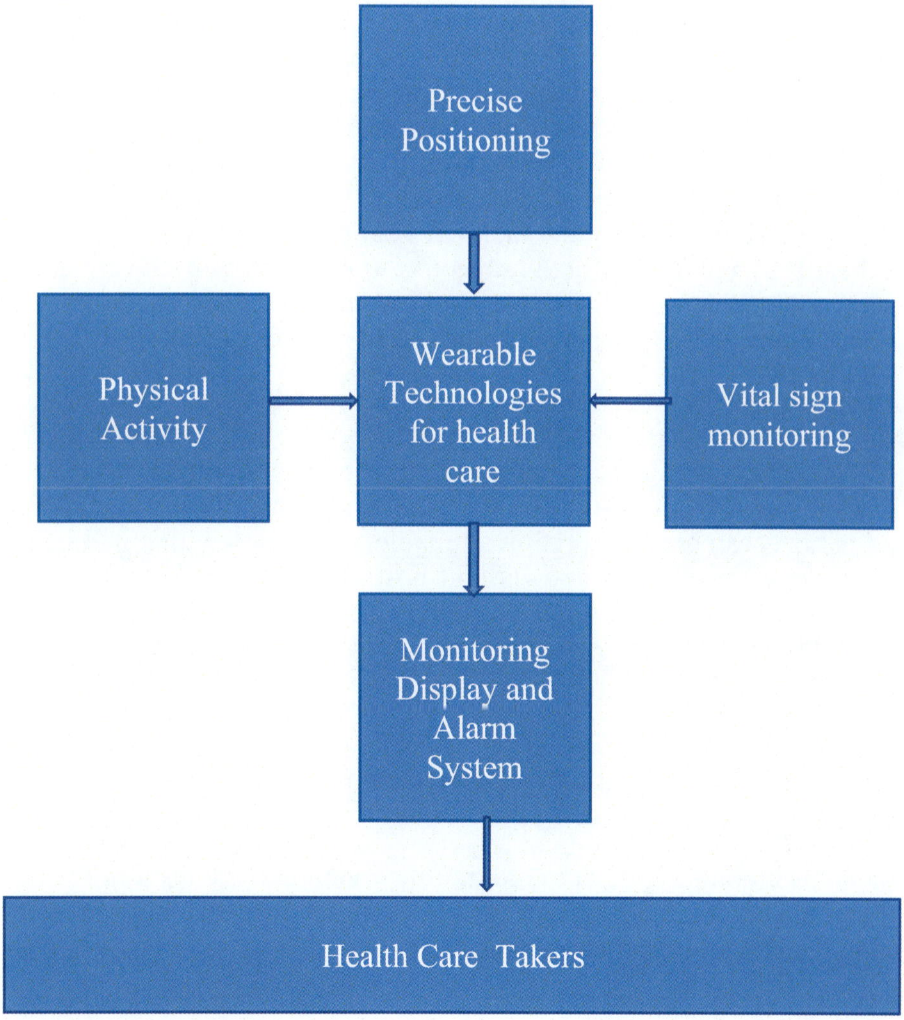

Fig. (5). Design of wearable device of adults.

Self-Tracking and Monitoring

PRO model enables the patient to be proactive and also they can decide on what they are doing. This can be done by having the patient's self-report which would be in a descriptive manner and in subjective manner. However this method would be inconsistent and unreliable when objective measures are to be made as part of the monitoring. Furthermore, telemonitoring monitors data passively and then send the data to patient and their provider. Reports of PRO models are in the form of subjective data, whereas telemonitoring monitors objective data in the quantifiable variables. QSH model monitors both quantifiable and non-quantifiable variables. QSH model facilitates patients with a better understanding of their health by combining both subjective symptoms with objective criteria. The majority of smart wearable sensors follow telemonitoring model, but only a few models allow the user to input subjective and objective data.

Patients with chronic diseases can be monitored remotely, and it is the best way to monitor daily routine activities. Patients need not to be in hospital for a long duration, and they should be discharged, thereby continuing to monitor their condition on their own. In this way, we can gather more authentic and accurate data and patients can be monitored in a reliable way remotely that will help them in the cost management associated with the hospital stay.

Cardiopulmonary and vascular monitoring devices exist, which monitors by implanting wireless devices and sending reports to the smartphone. Patients have 24 hours of access to the smartphone to monitor the report. Most of the devices are external and can be placed around the wrist or thorax to accurately monitor cardiac function. Some multimodal sensors monitor respiratory rates, oxygen saturation, coughing events, and other respiratory variables.

Glucose home monitoring devices monitor the blood glucose level of the patients using wearable devices, greatly increasing the self-confidence of the patient and improving the ability in diabetic management.

The evolution of smart wearable sensor devices and their capability of self-monitoring, tracking, and indicating health parameters and symptoms have brought a great revolution in the health care system and change in the attitude of patients.

Furthermore, pervasive networks [54, 55] can assist residents by providing memory support, remote control of household appliances, medical data look-up, automatic medication dispensing, and emergency communications and services.

The pandemic situation has changed the way of living, with working from home as a new norm, thus being able to work from anywhere in the world. This has led to migration from urban to rural locality. Smart wearable devices can access and administer medical aid remotely, helping the aging population live in the rural environment without worrying about medical assistance. Smart wearable devices with sensors and integration of the Internet of things will take health care treatment to the next level, and timely assistance could enable reaching people in rural areas also.

With the advancements in wearable technology and IoT, it should be possible for older adults [56] to live independently. Researchers are focusing on designing smart health care systems which can ensure remote monitoring of elders and alert the medical practitioners in case of emergency, making elders more independent. It is also the need of the hour, as it was observed during the peak outbreak of the pandemic that elders who lived on their own were not able to access the required medical assistance.

While developing the applications, we need to keep in mind that recommendations by medical professionals are required at each stage of development, and it is difficult to get such recommendations. During the testing phase, monitoring systems do not use real-time data to check the efficacy of the system. There is an issue in getting expert's acceptability or performing clinical validation of the system/application developed. User-friendliness is another issue for both the patients and health care professionals.

The challenges faced in collecting high-quality data using WS and IoT applications sensors are motion artifacts, body movements, and respiration. Security and privacy of the data collected from patients are also challenging aspects. It has been reported that most of the wearable's accuracy is affected by the electromagnetic interference of power lines. There is a limitation of the availability of hardware for removing the noise, and hence there is a necessity to rely on software for removing noise. Moreover, common challenges in data collection and processing include data loss, buffering, network communication, monitoring, processing, and low signal [57] strength, transmission speed, and battery life.

Some of the challenges that are to be overcome while designing wearable infant health monitoring systems are accuracy, mode of communication and associated issues, the life span of the battery, size and comfortability of wearing the device, user-friendliness, flexibility, and reusability of the designed device.

CONCLUDING REMARKS

In the current scenario, there is a rapid advancement in information and communication technology. The implementation and deployment of these technologies have significant benefits in the health care domain. In this work, we have discussed integrating smart wearable sensors and IoT to enhance the automatic monitoring and alerting systems for health care improvement. In the healthcare domain, there are several challenges that need to be addressed before digitalizing the health care sector.

CONSENT FOR PUBLICATION

Not applicable.

CONFLICT OF INTEREST

The authors declare no conflict of interest, financial or otherwise.

ACKNOWLEDGEMENT

Declared none.

REFERENCES

[1] P. Mehrotra, "Biosensors and their applications – A review", *J. Oral Biol. Craniofac. Res.*, vol. 6, no. 2, pp. 153-159, 2016.
[http://dx.doi.org/10.1016/j.jobcr.2015.12.002] [PMID: 27195214]

[2] X.J. John, *Zhang and Kazunori Hoshino, "Molecular Sensors and Nanodevices, Principles, Designs and Application in Biomedical Engineering"*. Elsevier, 2014.

[3] Y.H. Tsou, X.Q. Zhang, H. Zhu, S. Syed, and X. Xu, "Drug delivery to the brain across the blood–brain barrier using nanomaterials", *Small,* vol. 14, no. 25, p. 1801588, 2018.
[http://dx.doi.org/10.1002/smll.201801588] [PMID: 29927551]

[4] L. Cheng, X. Wang, F. Gong, T. Liu, and Z. Liu, "2D nanomaterials for cancer theranostic applications", *Adv. Mater.,* vol. 32, no. 13, p. 1902333, 2020.
[http://dx.doi.org/10.1002/adma.201902333] [PMID: 31353752]

[5] W. Zhu, Z. Chen, Y. Pan, R. Dai, Y. Wu, Z. Zhuang, D. Wang, Q. Peng, C. Chen, and Y. Li, "Functionalization of hollow nanomaterials for catalytic applications: Nanoreactor construction", *Adv. Mater.,* vol. 31, no. 38, p. 1800426, 2019.
[http://dx.doi.org/10.1002/adma.201800426] [PMID: 30125990]

[6] https://www.treehugger.com/environmental-sensors-4858156

[7] Hatice Ceylan Koydemir and Aydogan Ozcan, "Wearable and Implantable Sensors for Biomedical Applications", *Annual Review of Analytical Chemistry,* vol. 11, pp. 6.1-6.20, 2018.

[8] P. Sorte, A. Golande, A. Yermalkar, V. Suryawanshi, U. Wanjare, and S. Satpute, "Smart Hospital for Heart Disease Prediction Using IOT", *International Journal of Innovative Technology and Exploring Engineering.,* vol. 8, no. 9, pp. 2278-3075, 2019.

[9] R.B. D'Agostino Sr, R.S. Vasan, M.J. Pencina, P.A. Wolf, M. Cobain, J.M. Massaro, and W.B. Kannel, "General cardiovascular risk profile for use in primary care: the Framingham Heart Study", *Circulation,* vol. 117, no. 6, pp. 743-753, 2008.
[http://dx.doi.org/10.1161/CIRCULATIONAHA.107.699579] [PMID: 18212285]

[10] P. Kakria, N.K. Tripathi, and P. Kitipawang, "A Real-Time Health Monitoring System for Remote Cardiac Patients Using Smartphone and Wearable Sensors", *Int. J. Telemed. Appl.,* vol. 2015, pp. 1-11, 2015.
[http://dx.doi.org/10.1155/2015/373474]

[11] J. Coughlan, and R. Manduchi, A mobile phone way finding system for visually impaired users.*Assistive Technology Research Series.,* vol. 25, p. 849, 2009.

[12] S.J. Lane, N.M. Heddle, E. Arnold, and I. Walker, "A review of randomized controlled trials comparing the effectiveness of hand held computers with paper methods for data collection", *BMC Med. Inform. Decis. Mak.*, vol. 6, no. 1, p. 23, 2006. [http://dx.doi.org/10.1186/1472-6947-6-23] [PMID: 16737535]

[13] M.N.K. Boulos, A. Anastasiou, E. Bekiaris, and M. Panou, "Geo-enabled technologies for independent living: Examples from four European projects", *Technol. Disabil.*, vol. 23, no. 1, pp. 7-17, 2011. [http://dx.doi.org/10.3233/TAD-2011-0300]

[14] C. Free, G. Phillips, L. Felix, L. Galli, V. Patel, and P. Edwards, "The effectiveness of M-health technologies for improving health and health services: a systematic review protocol", *BMC Res. Notes,* vol. 3, no. 1, p. 250, 2010. [http://dx.doi.org/10.1186/1756-0500-3-250] [PMID: 20925916]

[15] S. Patel, H. Park, P. Bonato, L. Chan, and M. Rodgers, "A review of wearable sensors and systems with application in rehabilitation", *J. Neuroeng. Rehabil.,* vol. 9, no. 1, p. 21, 2012. [http://dx.doi.org/10.1186/1743-0003-9-21] [PMID: 22520559]

[16] A. Kailas, Chia-Chin Chong, and F. Watanabe, "From mobile phones to personal wellness dashboards", *IEEE Pulse,* vol. 1, no. 1, pp. 57-63, 2010. [http://dx.doi.org/10.1109/MPUL.2010.937244] [PMID: 20875965]

[17] J. Kim, G.A. Salvatore, H. Araki, A.M. Chiarelli, Z. Xie, A. Banks, X. Sheng, Y. Liu, J.W. Lee, K.I. Jang, S.Y. Heo, K. Cho, H. Luo, B. Zimmerman, J. Kim, L. Yan, X. Feng, S. Xu, M. Fabiani, G. Gratton, Y. Huang, U. Paik, and J.A. Rogers, "Battery-free, stretchable optoelectronic systems for wireless optical characterization of the skin", *Sci. Adv.,* vol. 2, no. 8, p. e1600418, 2016. [http://dx.doi.org/10.1126/sciadv.1600418] [PMID: 27493994]

[18] N. Bhalla, P. Jolly, N. Formisano, and P. Estrela, "Introduction to biosensors", *Essays Biochem.,* vol. 60, no. 1, pp. 1-8, 2016. [http://dx.doi.org/10.1042/EBC20150001] [PMID: 27365030]

[19] K. Meddah, M. Kedir Talha, M. Bahoura, and H. Zairi, "FPGA-based system for heart rate monitoring", *IET Circuits Dev. Syst.,* vol. 13, no. 6, pp. 771-782, 2019. [http://dx.doi.org/10.1049/iet-cds.2018.5204]

[20] G.V. Angelov, D.P. Nikolakov, I.N. Ruskova, E.E. Gieva and M.L. Spasova, "Healthcare Sensing and Monitoring", Enhanced Living Environments, Lecture Notes in Computer Science, Springer, Vol. 11369, pp. 226-262, 2019.

[21] B.W. An, J.H. Shin, S.Y. Kim, J. Kim, S. Ji, J. Park, Y. Lee, J. Jang, Y.G. Park, E. Cho, S. Jo, and J.U. Park, "Smart Sensor Systems for Wearable Electronic Devices", *Polymers (Basel),* vol. 9, no. 12, p. 303, 2017. [http://dx.doi.org/10.3390/polym9080303] [PMID: 30970981]

[22] M. Jacob Rodrigues, O. Postolache, and F. Cercas, "Physiological and Behavior Monitoring Systems for Smart Healthcare Environments: A Review", *Sensors (Basel),* vol. 20, no. 8, p. 2186, 2020. [http://dx.doi.org/10.3390/s20082186] [PMID: 32290639]

[23] Z.H.K. Chong, Y.X. Tee, L.J. Toh, S.J. Phang, J.Y. Liew, B. Queck, and S. Gottipati, *Predicting Potential Alzheimer Medical Condition in Elderly Using IOT Sensors—Case Study,* 2017.https://ink. library.smu.edu.sg/sis_research/3834

[24] C. Lai Kwan, Y. Mahdid, R. Motta Ochoa, K. Lee, M. Park, and S. Blain-Moraes, "Wearable Technology for Detecting Significant Moments in Individuals with Dementia", *BioMed Res. Int.,* vol. 2019, pp. 1-13, 2019. [http://dx.doi.org/10.1155/2019/6515813] [PMID: 31662986]

[25] S. Khojasteh, J. Villar, C. Chira, V. González, and E. de la Cal, "Improving fall detection using an on-wrist wearable accelerometer", *Sensors (Basel),* vol. 18, no. 5, p. 1350, 2018. [http://dx.doi.org/10.3390/s18051350] [PMID: 29701721]

[26] S. Amendola, R. Lodato, S. Manzari, C. Occhiuzzi, and G. Marrocco, "RFID Technology for IoT-Based Personal Healthcare in Smart Spaces", *IEEE Internet Things J.,* vol. 1, no. 2, pp. 144-152, 2014. [http://dx.doi.org/10.1109/JIOT.2014.2313981]

[27] L Stevan Jr, "Sensors for Health Monitoring Sergio", *Scholarly Community Encyclopedia Accessed on.,* 2021.

[28] B. Zhang, J. Ren, Y. Cheng, B. Wang, and Z. Wei, "Health Data Driven on Continuous Blood Pressure Prediction Based on Gradient Boosting Decision Tree Algorithm", *IEEE Access,* vol. 7, pp. 32423-32433, 2019.
[http://dx.doi.org/10.1109/ACCESS.2019.2902217]

[29] G. Appelboom, E. Camacho, M.E. Abraham, S.S. Bruce, E.L.P. Dumont, B.E. Zacharia, R. D'Amico, J. Slomian, J.Y. Reginster, O. Bruyère, and E.S. Connolly Jr, "Smart wearable body sensors for patient self-assessment and monitoring", *Arch. Public Health,* vol. 72, no. 1, p. 28, 2014.
[http://dx.doi.org/10.1186/2049-3258-72-28] [PMID: 25232478]

[30] L.K. Simone, N. Sundarrajan, X. Luo, Y. Jia, and D.G. Kamper, "A low cost instrumented glove for extended monitoring and functional hand assessment", *J. Neurosci. Methods,* vol. 160, no. 2, pp. 335-348, 2007.
[http://dx.doi.org/10.1016/j.jneumeth.2006.09.021] [PMID: 17069892]

[31] S. Bouwstra, W. Chen, L. Feijs, and S. Bambang-Oetomo, "Smart Jacket Design for Neonatal Monitoring with Wearable Sensors", *Proceedings of 6th International Workshop on Wearable and Implantable Body Sensor Networks* pp. 162-167, 2009.
[http://dx.doi.org/10.1109/BSN.2009.40]

[32] S.F. Memon, M. Memon, and S. Bhatti, "Wearable technology for infant health monitoring: a survey", *IET Circuits Dev. Syst.,* vol. 14, no. 2, pp. 115-129, 2020.
[http://dx.doi.org/10.1049/iet-cds.2018.5447]

[33] P. Vanhaesebrouck, K. Allegaert, J. Bottu, C. Debauche, H. Devlieger, M. Docx, A. François, D. Haumont, J. Lombet, J. Rigo, K. Smets, I. Vanherreweghe, B.V. Overmeire, P.V. Reempts, and P.V. Reempts, Extremely Preterm Infants in Belgium Study Group, "The EPIBEL study: outcomes to discharge from hospital for extremely preterm infants in Belgium", *Pediatrics,* vol. 114, no. 3, pp. 663-675, 2004.
[http://dx.doi.org/10.1542/peds.2003-0903-L] [PMID: 15342837]

[34] Y.C. Wu, P-F. Chen, Z.A. Hu, C.H. Chang, G.C. Lee, and W.C. Yu, "A mobile health monitoring system using RFID ring-type pulse sensor", *Proceeding of 8th IEEE International Conference of Dependable, Autonomic and Secure Computing* pp. 317-322, 2009.
[http://dx.doi.org/10.1109/DASC.2009.136]

[35] F.A. Rhoads, and J. Grandner, "Assessment of an aural infrared sensor for body temperature measurement in children", *Clin. Pediatr. (Phila.),* vol. 29, no. 2, pp. 112-115, 1990. [http://dx.doi.org/10.1177/000992289002900209] [PMID: 2302899]

[36] P.S. Pandian, K. Mohanavelu, K.P. Safeer, T.M. Kotresh, D.T. Shakunthala, P. Gopal, and V.C. Padaki, "Smart Vest: Wearable multi-parameter remote physiological monitoring system", *Med. Eng. Phys.,* vol. 30, no. 4, pp. 466-477, 2008.
[http://dx.doi.org/10.1016/j.medengphy.2007.05.014] [PMID: 17869159]

[37] M.R. Yuce, "Recent wireless body sensors: Design and implementation", *IEEE MTT-S International Microwave Workshop Series on RF and Wireless Technologies for Biomedical and Healthcare Applications (IMWS-BIO)* pp. 1-3, 2013.
[http://dx.doi.org/10.1109/IMWS-BIO.2013.6756254]

[38] M. Chan, D. Estève, J.Y. Fourniols, C. Escriba, and E. Campo, "Smart wearable systems: Current status and future challenges", *Artif. Intell. Med.,* vol. 56, no. 3, pp. 137-156, 2012.
[http://dx.doi.org/10.1016/j.artmed.2012.09.003] [PMID: 23122689]

[39] S. López-Soriano, and J. Parrón, "Wearable RFID tag antenna for healthcare applications", *Proceedings of IEEE-APS Topical Conference on Antennas and Propagation in Wireless Communications (APWC)* pp. 287-290, 2015. [http://dx.doi.org/10.1109/APWC.2015.7300156]

[40] X. Chang, X. Tang, L. Chen, A. Liu, and Y. Wang, *Na Liu, Yurong Wang, Hospital IoT big data and real-time monitoring and nursing intervention for patients with insomnia.* vol. Vol. 81. Microprocessors and Microsystems, 2021.

[41] M. Shankar Lingam, and G.S. Raghavendra, "Internet of Things (IoT) constructed Individual Healthcare in Smart Spaces through the RFID", *International Journal of Research and Analytical Reviews,* vol. 7, no. 2, pp. 549-555, 2020.

[42] S. Majumder, T. Mondal, and M. Deen, "Wearable Sensors for Remote Health Monitoring", *Sensors (Basel),* vol. 17, no. 12, p. 130, 2017. [http://dx.doi.org/10.3390/s17010130] [PMID: 28085085]

[43] A.M. Ngueleu, A.K. Blanchette, L. Bouyer, D. Maltais, B.J. McFadyen, H. Moffet, and C.S. Batcho, *Design and Accuracy of an Instrumented Insole Using Pressure Sensors for Step Count,* vol. 19, no. 984, 2019.

[44] T.G. Stavropoulos, A. Papastergiou, L. Mpaltadoros, S. Nikolopoulos, and I. Kompatsiaris, "IoT Wearable Sensors and Devices in Elderly Care: A Literature Review", *Sensors (Basel),* vol. 20, no. 10, p. 2826, 2020. [http://dx.doi.org/10.3390/s20102826] [PMID: 32429331]

[45] Z. Wang, Z. Yang, T. Dong, Z. Wang, Z. Yang, and T. Dong, "A Review of Wearable Technologies for Elderly Care that Can Accurately Track Indoor Position, Recognize Physical Activities and Monitor Vital Signs in Real Time", *Sensors (Basel),* vol. 17, no. 2, p. 341, 2017. [http://dx.doi.org/10.3390/s17020341] [PMID: 28208620]

[46] D. Rodrigues, F. Luis-Ferreira, J. Sarraipa, and R. Goncalves, "Behavioural Monitoring of Alzheimer Patients with Smartwatch Based System", *Proceedings of International Conference on Intelligent Systems* pp. 771-775, 2018. [http://dx.doi.org/10.1109/IS.2018.8710487]

[47] J. Sharma, and S. Kaur, "Gerontechnology - The study of alzheimer disease using cloud computing", *Proceedings of International Conference on Energy, Communication, Data Analytics and Soft Computing* pp. 3726-3733, 2017. [http://dx.doi.org/10.1109/ICECDS.2017.8390159]

[48] S.S. Aljehani, R.A. Alhazmi, S.S. Aloufi, B.D. Aljehani, and R. Abdulrahman, "iCare: Applying IoT Technology for Monitoring Alzheimer's Patients", *Proceedings of International Conference on Computer Applications & Information Security (ICCAIS) IEEE,* pp. 1–6, 2018. [http://dx.doi.org/10.1109/CAIS.2018.8442010]

[49] M. Karakaya, G. Sengül, and A. Bostan, "Remotely Monitoring Activities of the Elders Using Smart Watches", *International Journal of Scientific Research in Information Systems Engineering,* vol. 3, no. 1, pp. 56-60, 2017.

[50] S. Barri Khojasteh, J.R. Villar, E. de la Cal, V.M. González, J. Sedano, and H.R. Yazgan, "Evaluation of a Wrist-Based Wearable Fall Detection Method", *Proceedings of 13th International conference on Hybrid Artificial Intelligence Systems,* 2018pp. 377-386 [http://dx.doi.org/10.1007/978-3-319-92639-1_31]

[51] D.L. Algase, E.R.A. Beattie, S.A. Leitsch, and C.A. Beel-Bates, "Biomechanical activity devices to index wandering behaviour in dementia", *American Journal of Alzheimer Disease and other Dementias.,* vol. 18, no. 3, pp. 85-92, 2003. [http://dx.doi.org/10.1177/153331750301800202]

[52] R. Lu, Y. Xu, X. Li, Y. Fan, W. Zeng, Y. Tan, K. Ren, W. Chen, and X. Cao, " Evaluation of

Wearable Sensor Devices in Parkinson's Disease: A Review of Current Status and Future Prospects", *Parkinson's Disease.,* p. 8, 2020.

[53] G. Appelboom, E. Camacho, M.E. Abraham, S.S. Bruce, E.L.P. Dumont, B.E. Zacharia, R. D'Amico, J. Slomian, J.Y. Reginster, O. Bruyère, and E.S. Connolly Jr, "Smart wearable body sensors for patient self-assessment and monitoring", *Arch. Public Health,* vol. 72, no. 1, p. 28, 2014. [http://dx.doi.org/10.1186/2049-3258-72-28] [PMID: 25232478]

[54] Javier Andreu-Perez, "Daniel R. Leff, H.M.D. Ip, and Guang-Zhong Yang, "From Wearable Sensors to Smart Implants – Towards Pervasive and Personalised Healthcare"", *IEEE Trans. Biomed. Eng.,* vol. 62, no. 12, pp. 2750-2762, 2015. [http://dx.doi.org/10.1109/TBME.2015.2422751] [PMID: 25879838]

[55] B. Rubehn, C. Bosman, R. Oostenveld, P. Fries, and T. Stieglitz, "A MEMS-based flexible multichannel ECoG-electrode array", *J. Neural Eng.,* vol. 6, no. 3, p. 036003, 2009. [http://dx.doi.org/10.1088/1741-2560/6/3/036003] [PMID: 19436080]

[56] M.M. Baig, S. Afifi, H. GholamHosseini, and F. Mirza, "A Systematic Review of Wearable Sensors and IoT-Based Monitoring Applications for Older Adults – a Focus on Ageing Population and Independent Living", *J. Med. Syst.,* vol. 43, no. 8, p. 233, 2019. [http://dx.doi.org/10.1007/s10916-019-1365-7] [PMID: 31203472]

[57] N. Hegde, and E. Sazonov, "SmartStep: A fully integrated, low power insole monitor", *Electronics (Basel),* vol. 3, no. 2, pp. 381-397, 2014. [http://dx.doi.org/10.3390/electronics3020381]

SUBJECT INDEX

Sivakumar R., Dimiter Velev, Basim Alhadidi, S. Vidhya, Sheeja V. Francis and B. Prabadevi (Eds.)

E

F

G

H

I

L

M

N

O

P

R

S

T

V

W

Made in the USA
Las Vegas, NV
15 November 2026

6b5267fc-5b92-4db4-8919-29411c82f2edR01